MW00529789

WHEN DOCTORS SAY NO

MEDICAL ETHICS SERIES

DAVID H. SMITH AND ROBERT M. VEATCH, EDITORS

Norman L. Cantor. *Advance Directives and the Pursuit
of Death with Dignity*

Norman L. Cantor. *Legal Frontiers of Death and Dying*

Arthur L. Caplan. *Am I My Brother's Keeper?
Essays on the Ethical Frontiers of Biomedicine*

Arthur L. Caplan. *If I Were a Rich Man Could I Buy a Pancreas?
And Other Essays on the Ethics of Health Care*

James F. Childress. *Practical Reasoning in Bioethics:
Principles, Metaphors, and Analogies*

Cynthia B. Cohen, ed. *Casebook on the Termination
of Life-Sustaining Treatment and the Care of the Dying*

Cynthia B. Cohen, ed. *New Ways of Making Babies:
The Case of Egg Donation*

Roger B. Dworkin. *Limits: The Role of the Law
in Bioethical Decision Making*

Larry Gostin, ed. *Surrogate Motherhood: Politics and Privacy*

Christine Grady. *The Search for an AIDS Vaccine: Ethical Issues
in the Development and Testing of a Preventive HIV Vaccine*

A Report by the Hastings Center. *Guidelines on the Termination
of Life-Sustaining Treatment and the Care of the Dying*

Paul Lauritzen. *Pursuing Parenthood:
Ethical Issues in Assisted Reproduction*

Joanne Lynn, M.D., ed. *By No Extraordinary Means:
The Choice to Forgo Life-Sustaining Food and Water, Expanded Edition*

William F. May. *The Patient's Ordeal*

Richard W. Momeyer. *Confronting Death.*

Thomas H. Murray, Mark A. Rothstein, and Robert F. Murray, Jr., editors.
The Human Genome Project and the Future of Health Care

S. Kay Toombs, David Barnard, and Ronald Carson, eds. *Chronic Illness:
From Experience to Policy*

Robert M. Veatch. *The Patient as Partner:
A Theory of Human-Experimentation Ethics*

Robert M. Veatch. *The Patient-Physician Relation:
The Patient as Partner, Part 2*

Robert F. Weir, ed. *Physician-Assisted Suicide*

WHEN DOCTORS SAY NO

THE BATTLEGROUND
OF MEDICAL FUTILITY

SUSAN B. RUBIN

INDIANA UNIVERSITY PRESS
BLOOMINGTON AND INDIANAPOLIS

This book is a publication of

Indiana University Press

601 North Morton Street

Bloomington, Indiana 47404-3797 USA

www.indiana.edu/~iupress

Telephone orders   800-842-6796

Fax orders   812-855-7931

Orders by e-mail   iuporder@indiana.edu

The paper used in this publication meets the minimum requirements of American National Standard for Information Sciences—Permanence of Paper for Printed Library Materials, ANSI Z39.48-1984.

Manufactured in the United States of America

Library of Congress Cataloging-in-Publication Data

Rubin, Susan B., date

When doctors say No : the battleground of medical futility / Susan B. Rubin.

p.   cm. — (Medical ethics series)

Includes bibliographical references and index.

ISBN 0-253-33463-2 (alk. paper)

1. Medical ethics.   2. Therapeutics—Decision making—Moral and ethical aspects.   3. Care of the sick—Decision making—Moral and ethical aspects.   I. Title.   II. Series.

R725.5.R83   1998

174'.2—dc21   98-6798

1   2   3   4   5   03   02   01   00   99   98

❖ TO MY FAMILY, ❖
BOTH GIVEN AND CREATED

CONTENTS

ACKNOWLEDGMENTS

No ONE THINKS, creates, or lives well in isolation. And thankfully I've had to do none of these. To the contrary, I've been blessed with a close circle of friends, family, and colleagues. For their ongoing presence and participation in my life, I am forever grateful.

For teaching me much about the value of family, the meaning of health, illness, and resiliency, and the importance both of having a good heart and being my own person, I want to acknowledge and thank my mother and grandmother, Sharon Rubin and Rose Winer, as well as my brothers Mark and David Rubin. I give thanks to them, and to my father and his wife, Leonard and Charlene Rubin, for their support.

When it comes to undertaking a project like this, one could not pick a better muse. For her willingness to engage in lively debate at a moment's notice, her consistently insightful comments, her critical contribution to my thinking, and her involvement in every stage of the project, I want to thank in particular Esther Wagner, a natural-born philosopher.

A number of other individuals tirelessly read various drafts of this manuscript, offering detailed comments that honed my thinking and substantially improved the finished product. In particular, Robert Veatch, LeRoy Walters, and John Lantos offered invaluable insights every step of the way, helped me to strengthen and sharpen the argument, and served as a source of real guidance. Carol Bayley read everything and offered unwavering support and important comments throughout. Leigh Raymond read the entire manuscript in record time and offered cogent and valuable suggestions. My first-class editors at Indiana University Press, Robert Sloan and Michael Nelson, were a pleasure to work with and made excellent suggestions that clearly improved the book. And the exceptional librarians at the

National Reference Center for Bioethics Literature at the Kennedy Institute of Ethics at Georgetown University generously helped at many steps along the way with all of the little but critically important details.

Thanks go as well to my trusted colleague, Laurie Zoloth-Dorfman, for being a genuine ally in this debate and for always expanding and enriching my perspective. I am further indebted to the clinicians and ethics committees whose experience and deeply held convictions refined my thoughts about futility. I thank them for sharing their stories and for consistently teaching me so much.

For their overall support, reliably good humor, and irreplaceable assistance at critical junctures, I want especially to thank Mark Rubin and Rachel Wagner. For keeping things in perspective and lifting my spirits in between rewrites, I want to thank Laura Stuchinsky, Paula Taubman, Laurie Silverman, Betty Mayo, Teresa Blaydes Raymond, Joy Riggs, Jackie Bocian, Cat Myser, Jeff Kahn, Gary Foster, Bill Reichle, Tony Muniz, and Zachary Harris.

WHEN DOCTORS SAY NO

❖   1   ❖
_____

WHOSE FACTS, WHOSE VALUES?
An Overview of the Futility Debate

A DILEMMA HAS captured the attention of health care professionals, patients, families, insurers, public policy analysts, and ethicists alike. It has arisen in response to the so-called problem of medical futility and finds its expression in the queries of physicians who ask, "If this treatment is futile, can't we just stop? Can't we just say no?"

This book is an attempt to answer their question, to critique both the concept of futility and the structure of the debate that surrounds appeals to futility in medical decision making, and finally to point the way towards a much needed, more defensible, and more fruitful line of inquiry.

The underlying question is a deceptively simple one: Should physicians be empowered to make unilateral medical decisions on the basis of futility? In other words, should physicians' opinions about the futility of a particular treatment be sufficient to justify their refusal to offer, provide or continue treatment that patients expressly desire?

In what follows, I will examine critically the nature and limit of the futility appeals made most frequently in the clinical setting and consider whether they are sufficient to justify physician unilateral decision making. In the end I will argue that no current formulation of futility is sufficient to justify physician unilateral decision making and that the use of the concept should be abandoned. In perhaps my most distinctive contribution to the debate, I will apply a social constructionist theory of knowledge to uncover and challenge the presumptions underlying the standard approach to futility judgments. I will also argue that the rhetoric of futility has distracted and deflected our attention and obscured the very issues most in need of considered public reflection and debate. Finally, I will consider the clinical and public policy implications of my argument and discuss some alternative responses available to a physician tempted to refuse to offer, provide, or continue treatment on the grounds of futility.

It is necessary to clarify my frame of reference and use of terms. I have deliberately focussed on futility conflicts that arise in the context of the individual physician-patient relationship because that is the paradigmatic example most thoroughly discussed to date in the literature, in the clinical setting, and at the institutional and public policy level. But other involved parties, such as non-physician health care professionals, family members or other surrogates, insurers, and even society at large have no less an important stake in the futility debate. In fact, much of what I say has significance beyond the individual physician-patient encounter.

Accordingly, the words "patient" and "physician" should be understood throughout to encompass far more than the individual patient and the individual physician in an individual medical encounter. For example, when a patient is incapable of participating in the decision making process, family members or other surrogate decision makers might find themselves facing conflicts over futility when they act on the patient's behalf. In such instances, one could substitute the words "family members" or "surrogate decision makers" for "patient." To avoid overly cumbersome prose, I intend the word "patient" to be read inclusively throughout, encompassing all such possibilities. Likewise, the wide range of health care professionals involved in any patient's care might find themselves facing conflicts over futility. And further, it may be the medical profession's and not just the individual physician's assessment of appropriate behavior that is at stake in a conflict over futility. Again, to simplify the linguistics of my argument, I intend the term "physician" to be read inclusively as well, encompassing both non-physician health care professionals and the medical profession generally when appropriate.

This being said, my use of terms should not be misinterpreted to imply that the patient's interests and perspective will always be in harmony with the family's or surrogate decision maker's interests and perspective, that the individual physician's interests and perspective will always be shared by their peers, or that all potential conflicts are reducible to the physician-patient conflict. Clearly potential conflicts may exist not only between physicians and their patients, but also between patients and family members or other surrogate decision makers, between patients and their insurers, between patients and the larger society, among members of the health care team, between members of the health care team and family members or other surrogates, between members of the health care team and insurers, between the health care community and the larger society, and within the larger society. The complicated web of relationships converging in any given medical encounter inevitably expands the range of potential conflicts.

This book begins with an analysis of the paradigmatic conflict between physicians and patients in order to specify concretely what is at stake in the futility debate and in any futility conflict. Then, to situate the debate in its broader context, I consider the relationship between the medical profession and society, and the specific roles each plays in addressing the concerns outlined in this book. By extension, my discussion addresses many of the concerns particular to other stakeholders such as family members, other surrogate decision makers, non-physician health care professionals, and insurers. A central framing question concerns standing: Who among the various stakeholders should have the authority to make which kinds of decisions? In the course of this book I consider this question at the level of the individual encounter, as well as at the level of institutional and public policy.

At its heart the futility debate is a debate about power: who should have it, and how it should be exercised. Not insignificantly, the debate is taking place in an era characterized by an increasingly competitive health care marketplace, a rise in managed care, growing attention to cost and the demands of the bottom line, and heightened interest in the standardization of medical practice. As a result, the stakes of the futility debate are important not only for health care professionals and patients, but for the broader society as well. At issue is the very meaning and place of medicine in society, and the scope of authority that society grants to health care professionals.

Given the diverse range of concerns surrounding the futility debate, it is necessary to be clear about the limited focus of this book. This is not a book about the broad problem of the need to set limits in medicine, to ensure the just allocation of our health care resources, to prioritize our needs, to contain or reduce costs, to improve efficiency, or to reform the health care system. Rather, this book offers an extended examination of the specific proposal that limits be set on the basis of medical judgments of so-called futility. Unquestionably, limits can and should be set in medical encounters. At issue in this book is whether futility can ever be a defensible ground for such limit setting.

An Introduction to the Debate

The appeal to futility as a justification for withholding or withdrawing treatment, even against the express wishes of patients, has gained tremendous popularity in the clinical setting[1] and medical literature. The appeal is generally grounded in the widespread conviction that physicians are not obligated to provide, and patients do not have a right to receive, medically futile treatment.

The strength of this increasingly popular conviction and the frequency with which it is now expressed in the clinical context marks a significant shift in the paradigm case of end-of-life decision making in bioethics and has ushered in a new era of clinical dilemmas. While the older paradigm arose from a clash between patients who wanted to "say no" to medical interventions and health care professionals who wanted to "do everything possible" despite patient resistance, the newer paradigm arises from precisely the opposite conflict: a clash between patients who want "everything possible" done and health care professionals who want to "say no" to medical interventions they deem futile.

But while there is a fairly clear ethical and legal framework for understanding and responding to the older paradigm case of bioethics, a framework for the newer paradigm case of futility is still emerging. Though there is a growing body of literature on the use of the concept of futility to set limits, the concept itself, and the debate surrounding it, have yet to be the subject of a sufficiently thorough and critical conceptual analysis. This book advances the discussion by offering a new perspective on the structure and meaning of the futility debate and by underscoring the need for a new and more direct approach to the real problems underlying conflicts over futility.

The contemporary debate on the appropriate meaning and application of the concept of futility has been framed in several fundamentally mistaken ways. First, a potentially misleading philosophical analogy—the fact/value distinction—has been used to organize the variety of meanings ascribed to the notion of futility. Second, undefended presumptions have been made in favor of the nearly universal tendency to draw different conclusions about the normative weight of futility judgments depending on whether they are more factually or evaluatively based. Third, proposals for physician unilateral decision making as an answer to the identified conflict between physicians and their patients have given the debate a misguided focus and tone. I will comment briefly on each of these presumptions in turn.

The Fact/Value Distinction

Regardless of the normative position they endorse, nearly all participants in the futility debate share an acceptance, albeit oftentimes implicit, of the fact/value distinction as a rough way of contrasting different senses of futility. Considering the difficulty of formulating a single universally

applicable definition of futility, what is remarkable about the futility literature is not that attempts have been made to categorize different senses of futility, but rather that the results have been so uniformly consistent on both
sides of the debate.

In the standard analysis, the concept of futility is understood to have at
least two broad meanings, depending upon whether it is more substantially
an evaluative or factual judgment. This is not to say that all contributors to
the debate assume that all futility judgments must be either exclusively factually or exclusively evaluatively based. In fact, since it has increasingly been
suggested that even so-called factual judgments of futility have an evaluative component, the distinction is not being used as rigidly as it once was.[2]
Nonetheless, the futility debate remains guided by the notion that futility
judgments, and the conflicts that arise from them, seem sometimes more
driven by values and sometimes more by facts.

Accordingly, when futility operates as a primarily evaluative judgment,
it is understood to mean that a treatment is inappropriate because it would
just not be worth it. When futility operates as a primarily factual judgment, it is understood to mean that a treatment is ineffective because it
would just not work. I call these two different kinds of futility judgments
evaluative futility and factual or physiologic futility respectively to under-
score the influence that the fact/value distinction has had in organizing the
debate.[3]

Because the fact/value distinction has so significantly influenced the
structure and nature of the futility debate, I will use it as a way of deconstructing the different kinds of arguments represented in the literature. But
as will become evident, my initial application of the distinction will be only
as a heuristic or organizing device, not as an endorsement of the distinction
itself or its use in the futility debate. In fact, I will ultimately argue that the
fact/value distinction cannot be sustained, and so neither can the standard
normative distinction between factual or physiologic futility and evaluative
futility.

Shifting Obligations

The presumption that some futility judgments are based on value-free
scientific facts while others are based on value-laden opinions has supported
the nearly universal practice of according different normative weight to
judgments of physiologic and evaluative futility. In fact, most contributors to the futility debate rely on the fact/value distinction to draw different

normative conclusions depending on which kind of futility judgment is at issue.

The popular approach has been to acknowledge the selection of values to be primarily, if not exclusively, in the patient's domain and to assume the interpretation of facts to be primarily, if not exclusively, in the clinician's domain. Of course, not all commentators accept this distinction as defined. In fact, some would assign to physicians the latitude both to interpret the facts and to select the values according to which potential treatments would be selected.[4] But for the most part, contributors to the debate rely on the fact/value distinction to defend a different division of labor.

From this perspective, a tentative framework for decision making about potentially futile treatments has evolved, and gone without further challenge. This framework takes seriously the role of patients in making value judgments about the worth, desirability, and appropriateness of treatments their physicians identify as medically acceptable. And in most interpretations, the framework acknowledges the role society may have in limiting the availability of certain kinds of treatments.[5] But the framework just as clearly delineates a category of treatments with respect to which patient value judgments about worth and desirability are considered irrelevant: namely, treatments that have been deemed ineffective or physiologically futile.

According to the popular strategy of making an exception of physiologic futility, physicians' obligations to their patients are thought to shift depending on the sense in which treatments are judged to be futile.[6] Significantly, it has been assumed that physicians have a stronger obligation to provide treatments that they, in opposition to their patients, deem evaluatively futile, than to provide treatments that they, in opposition to their patients, deem physiologically futile.

Early evidence of the now popular approach to futility judgments, the prominence of the fact/value distinction, and the view that physicians' obligations shift depending upon the type of futility at issue can be found in a number of important documents, including the Hastings Center's 1987 *Guidelines on the Termination of Life-Sustaining Treatment and the Care of the Dying*. In a section on futility, the *Guidelines* explain:

> In the event that the patient or surrogate requests a treatment that the responsible health care professional regards as clearly futile in achieving its physiological objective and so offering no physiological benefit to the

patient, the professional has no obligation to provide it. However, the health care professional's value judgment that although a treatment will produce physiological benefit, the benefit is not sufficient to warrant the treatment, should not be used as a basis for determining a treatment to be futile.[7]

The Hastings Center Task Force, consistent with the thinking of the time, deliberately limited the authoritative scope of professional futility judgments. While health care professionals' judgments of physiologic futility justify foregoing treatment requested by patients, their evaluative judgments of the treatment's worth do not warrant provider refusal.

An influential 1988 article by Stuart Youngner entitled "Who Defines Futility?" bolstered the Hastings Center's stance and further solidified what has since become the popular approach to the problem of futility. He claimed,

> Physicians are in the best position to know the empirical facts about the many aspects of futility. I would argue, however, that *all, except for physiological futility* and an absolute inability to postpone death, also involve value judgments. . . . Physicians should not offer treatments that are physiologically futile or certain not to prolong life. . . . Beyond that, they run the risk of "giving opinions disguised as data."[8]

At issue in each of these documents, and in most of the literature that followed from them, is the nature and scope of expertise and the relationship between facts and values. Consistent with the Hastings Center's *Guidelines*, Youngner makes an exceptional case of physiological futility. In all cases but physiological futility, treatment decisions properly belong to patients because they involve personal value judgments about which only patients are expert. But in cases of physiological futility, treatment decisions properly belong to physicians because they involve factual scientific judgments about which only physicians are expert.

According to this model, for a patient's evaluative judgment to have relevance, let alone decisive weight, the treatment in question must qualify first on physiologic medical grounds. Echoing this sentiment, Allan S. Brett and Laurence B. McCullough offer a complementary explanation:

> [T]he foundation of the clinical encounter is a specified body of knowledge and expertise about what is beneficial for patients. When a patient seeks to exercise a positive right to an intervention, a necessary condition is that there is either an established or a theoretical medical basis for the patient's request. If that necessary condition has been satisfied, the patient's unique

circumstances and stated reasons for wanting the intervention should guide the final decision-making process.[9]

Under this widely accepted approach, if there is a medical basis for a patient request, i.e., if the treatment is not physiologically futile, then patient values have relevance and possibly even definitive weight. But if the treatment fits under the exceptional case of physiologic futility, then patient values are rendered irrelevant and physician unilateral refusal is justified.

Lawrence J. Schneiderman and Nancy S. Jecker offer a twist to this standard approach to specifying the conditions of physician obligation. Like Brett and McCullough, they begin with assumptions about the appropriate goals of medicine. For them, the aim of medicine must be to benefit patients as whole persons, not merely to produce desired physiologic effects. For a patient's judgment to have relevance, let alone decisive weight, the intervention in question must be sufficiently likely to provide a benefit worth pursuing *from the perspective of medicine.* In their specific formulation, this precludes treatments that have failed to work in the last 100 cases (what they term quantitatively futile treatments), or treatments that will result in creating total dependence on intensive medical care or permanent unconsciousness (what they term qualitatively futile treatments.)[10] What is notably different about the Schneiderman and Jecker approach is their claim that physicians as a group should have the authority to specify the conditions of futility not only in the factual realm, but in the evaluative realm as well.

A careful analysis of the literature reveals that nearly all contributors to the futility debate appeal to the fact/value distinction to justify drawing different normative conclusions depending upon the kind of futility judgment in question. There are, however, the exceptional few who draw the same normative conclusion regardless of the nature of the futility judgment. I will refer to the former approach as the standard analysis and to the latter as the more radical proposal. I argue that either approach as currently formulated is destined to fail. The standard analysis, representing the more modest proposal, fails because, as I will demonstrate, the fact/value distinction cannot be sustained, and so neither can the practice of making an exception of physiologic futility. The more radical proposal fails because, although it acknowledges the unavoidable existence of an evaluative component in all futility judgments, it unjustifiably stipulates and privileges as normative the medical profession's evaluative perspective.[11]

Departing from both approaches, I argue that since a conflict of values is ultimately and fundamentally at issue in any futility conflict, the only defensible resolution lies in directly confronting and debating the values at stake, not in merely stipulating the superiority of one particular set of values. For this reason I call for a specific kind of social discourse in which the competing values themselves can be evaluated and the acceptable terms of the relationship between the medical profession and society at large can be considered. The only evaluative decisions physicians can justifiably impose on patients are those that have been socially considered and sanctioned. Defending decisions because they are in accordance with *a priori* stipulated goals, practice standards, or position statements that are generated exclusively by the medical profession is not sufficient.

Unilateral Decision Making

Not only have the fact/value distinction and the related notion of shifting physician obligations gained popular acceptance as shared underlying assumptions for nearly all contributors to the futility debate, but the literature has also constructed unilateral decision making as the central battleground on which the moral legitimacy of physician refusal is fought. In a sense, the proposal of unilateral decision making follows logically as a subsequent assumption in the debate. If there is a substantive difference between physiologic and evaluative futility, namely that physiologic futility is devoid of the kind of evaluative content to which patients might otherwise have rights of authorship, if physician obligations shift depending upon whether treatment is physiologically or evaluatively futile, and if physicians are in the best position to recognize physiologic futility, then, the popular approach suggests, might not physician unilateral decision making based on physiologic futility be justified?

Proposals for physician unilateral decision making have taken a variety of forms in the futility debate. As sanctioned by influential professional position statments and promoted by many leading articles in the debate, physician unilateral decision making typically means not only that a physician need not obtain a patient's consent to forego a particular treatment, but also that the physician need not even discuss the decision to forego treatment with the patient. By designating the decision making as "unilateral," ultimate decision making authority is assigned exclusively to the physician, who in turn has no obligation to involve the patient in the process. Proposals favoring this approach to decision making are not uniformly representative of the pro-futility position, and in fact have been rejected by some of the strongest proponents of futility. But this extreme, albeit most problematic form of the appeal to futility has unquestionably been influential in shaping the subsequent debate.

The key to unilateral decision making is the assumption that the decision about how to proceed rests exclusively with the physician precisely because the decision is understood to be an exclusively medical one. Two classic modifications have been offered to the original formulation of "unilateral." First, it has been suggested that while physicians need not gain patient consent to forego treatment on the grounds of futility, they should always inform patients of their intentions and engage them in conversation. Second, it has been argued that only the medical profession (or some subset of it), and never the lone individual physician, should be empowered to judge unilaterally which interventions are futile and can thus be foregone without patient consent.

But I contend that with or without these modifications, the end result is essentially the same. Still at stake are the questions of who should be the ultimate authority in the physician-patient relationship and who should have the ultimate power to control the course of medical decision making. And on these questions, the pro-futility position remains uniform. In fact, even for those proponents of futility who insist upon full disclosure before physicians act either on their own or on their profession's judgment of futility, the substance and form of the recommended disclosure typically resembles a monologue rather than a dialogue. Even though these modified proposals recommend that the physician put the patient on notice, the bottom line is that the physician is given authority to act on the basis of futility, even against the objections of the patient. Regardless of the specific form physician unilateral decision making takes, then, the resultant decision making remains unilateral and not bilateral. For that reason, I will use the term "physician unilateral decision making" inclusively to describe the full range of proposals under which physicians are given ultimate and definitive authority to impose their judgments on patients.

The well-documented preoccupation with unilateral decision making as an answer to the identified conflict between physicians and their patients has shaped the futility debate in some unfortunate ways. By discouraging rather than encouraging genuine dialogue in the face of seemingly intractable conflict, unilateral decision making and its underlying assumptions threaten to obscure the issues and positions most at stake in the futility debate and most in need of critical examination.

One of the most striking features about the otherwise diverse futility literature is the essential uniformity of the basic orienting assumptions I have described. But the literature is remarkable for the insufficiently critical attention it has given to assumptions about the actual nature of futility judgments.[12] Are futility judgments factual or evaluative? Is there a philosophically sustainable difference between factual claims and value claims in the clinical setting? Are there any value-free factual scientific claims? What is the relationship between substantially factual and substantially evaluative judgments? Is the fact/value distinction really applicable? In what areas are physicians and patients expert? What should follow normatively from that expertise? Should the nature of physician obligations shift depending on the nature of the futility claim? Is unilateral decision making a morally defensible normative solution? These critical questions, which have yet to be addressed seriously or adequately in the futility literature, motivate my own investigation of the problem of futility.

The Context of the Futility Debate

It is helpful to understand the context of the futility debate before moving to a direct consideration of the deepest questions it raises. While the futility debate marks a shift in the paradigm case of bioethics, it is not the first time we have recognized or faced our medical and human limitations. Further, the contemporary futility debate did not introduce the ultimate question raised by the reality of limitations, that is, how we ought respond in the face of them. What the contemporary futility debate has introduced, and urged us to institutionalize, is a specific kind of answer, a particular kind of response to the reality of our acknowledged limitations: physician unilateral decision making. To situate the futility debate in its historical context, I will review the range of answers that have been offered over time to the reality of our limitations.

Historical Roots of Modern Medicine's Response to Limitation

Thus far I have suggested that the current futility debate marks a shift not only in the paradigm case of end-of-life decision making in bioethics, but also in our response to the reality of our own limitations. But it is important to recognize that the proposal of physician unilateral decision making in response to the limits of medicine did not appear on the scene *de novo*. In fact, the seeds for the futility debate were planted as far back as ancient Greece.

Both Plato and Hippocrates commented on the proper response of physicians and patients in the face of medical limitation. In each of their eras, excellent physicians were defined as those who refused to intervene when limitation had been reached, irrespective of patient desires or ability to pay. It was understood that the physician had a duty to withhold treatment when the application of the medical arts would be useless in curing long-standing sickness, healing underlying pathology, restoring function and productivity, improving quality of life, or forestalling death. The virtuous patient would not ask for medical intervention, but if he did, and even if he was extremely wealthy, the physician was obligated to refuse. As Plato describes Asclepius's practice of medicine:

> For those who were by nature and course of life sound of body but had some localized disease . . . [Asclepius] revealed the art of medicine . . . but . . . when bodies were diseased inwardly and throughout, he did not attempt by diet and by gradual evacuations and infusions to prolong a wretched existence for the man and have him beget in all likelihood similar wretched offspring. . . . [I]f a man was incapable of living in the established round and order of life, he did not think it worth while to treat him, since such a fellow is of no use either to himself or to the state.[13]

Following his example, Asclepius's sons practiced medicine similarly at Troy.

> They thought that the life of a man constitutionally sickly and intemperate was of no use to himself or others, and that the art of medicine should not be for such nor should they be given treatment even if they were richer than Midas.[14]

Taking a similar approach, Hippocrates counseled his students:

> Refuse to treat those who are overmastered by their diseases, realizing that in such cases medicine is powerless.[15]

Describing the proper response of patients, Hippocrates further elaborated:

> Whenever therefore a man suffers an illness which is too strong for the means at the disposal of medicine he surely must not expect that it can be overcome by medicine.[16]

Physicians in ancient Greece were obligated to have an appropriate sense of humility about what their art of medicine could offer. In most instances, their medicine was essentially powerless, and they were obligated to offer it only when it could genuinely cure or heal a patient.

In contrasting the practice of medicine in ancient Greece with today's practice, one recognizes immediately the vastly expanded knowledge, skill, technology, diagnostic and therapeutic procedures, and even pharmaceutical agents available to physicians today to augment their commitment to healing. Obviously, physicians in Plato's and Hippocrates' time were far more limited in what they could offer, and therefore in what they perceived to be their obligation towards patients in need. Accordingly, patients in ancient Greece were admonished to have far lower expectations of medicine than they could reasonably be asked to have today.

Given the nature and scope of medical practice today, the Greek texts may not seem as applicable and instructive as they once were. Nonetheless, these earliest undeveloped references to the problem of futility continue to inform the medical profession's understanding of its obligations in the face of limitation and are actually at the foundation of the contemporary futility debate.

Though indirect references to futility have a long history in the medical profession, only in the contemporary debate has the problem of futility become the object of extended explicit critical attention. As the debate has evolved, discussion has proceeded on several fronts with varying degrees of focus and precision. Explicit reference to the problem of futility, consideration of the moral weight that should be accorded to judgments of futility, and discussion of the proposal for physician unilateral decision making can be found in established guidelines for withholding and withdrawing treatment, in professional position statements, in institutional policies, and in case and statutory law. To provide the basis for the critical analysis that will follow, I will examine briefly the extent of the discussion of futility as it has emerged in each of these arenas.

Established Guidelines for Treatment Decisions

The emergence of the futility debate can be seen as a direct challenge to the generally established medical, ethical, and legal framework for treatment decisions. The general framework evolved first as a response to the challenge of finding ways to respect the capacity and right of patients in a beneficent therapeutic relationship to determine what happens to their bodies. Taking its bearings primarily from the principles[17] of beneficence, nonmaleficence, and autonomy, the framework puts forth different standards of decision making for different categories of patients.

The standard of informed consent and informed refusal is used for competent patients with decision making capacity as a way of acknowledging and respecting the capacity and right of autonomous individuals to participate in decision making about their bodies.

The standard of substituted judgment is used for formerly competent patients who no longer have decision making capacity as a way of continuing to respect the patient's right to participate in the decision making process. In order to gauge what the patient in this category would have wanted, we look for any directions the patient left and for a surrogate who can speak on behalf of the patient, from the perspective of her preferences, goals, and values.

Finally, the standard of best interest is used for the never or not yet competent patient, who never had decision making capacity, who does not yet have decision making capacity, or who lacks both capacity and an available surrogate. Because such patients cannot participate in the informed consent/informed refusal process, and because no one could legitimately claim to make a substituted judgment on their behalf, our only recourse is to contemplate what would be in their best interest by appealing to the principles of beneficence and nonmaleficence.

This established decision making framework has been written about and referenced extensively in the medical, ethical, and legal literature.[18] It has set the community standard for patient and surrogate involvement in medical decision making. But while the framework addresses the conditions that must be met to honor patient or surrogate refusal of proposed medical interventions, it does not address explicitly the conditions under which physicians can unilaterally refuse to provide treatments on the grounds of futility. One question raised by the futility debate, therefore, is whether similar or parallel guidelines can be crafted to allow for this kind of physician refusal. Influential documents like the previously mentioned Hastings Center's *Guidelines on the Termination of Life-Sustaining Treatment and the Care of the Dying* have moved in this direction, suggesting that futility might represent an important exception to the established framework, which otherwise provides for substantial patient and surrogate involvement in treatment decision making.

Professional Position Statements

The concept of futility has also received increasing attention from professional societies that have included discussions of futility and the limits of physician obligations in their position statements. Since the introduction of cardiopulmonary resuscitation (CPR) in the 1960s, there has been continuous discussion about whether to attempt or forego this procedure in a variety of patient situations. Because the do-not-resuscitate (DNR) decision has often served as a paradigm for decisions to withhold or withdraw other life sustaining treatments, it is not surprising that the evolving resuscitation literature parallels the growth of the contemporary futility debate.

Tracing the development of the resuscitation literature, we find the roots of the predominant view that resuscitation, like other medical therapies, is indicated in some situations and contraindicated in others. The American Heart Association's National Conferences on Cardiopulmonary Resuscitation and Emergency Cardiac Care in 1974, 1979, 1985, and 1992 all endorsed this view. According to the original intent behind the development of CPR, the 1974 conference guidelines explained,

> The purpose of CPR is the prevention of sudden, unexpected death. CPR is not indicated in certain situations, such as in cases of terminal irreversible illness where death is not unexpected.[19]

Contrary to this original intent, and in contrast to any other medical intervention, it is now routine for all hospitalized patients to receive CPR in the event of an arrest, unless a DNR order has been written in their charts. The presumption, in other words, is that resuscitation will automatically be attempted unless a decision to the contrary has been made and documented. For this reason discussions of indications and contraindications on the one hand, and discussions of the problem of futility on the other, have been on parallel tracks. The grounds upon which the medical profession has argued it is acceptable to judge CPR as contraindicated and to institute a DNR order have included irreversible brain death, patient refusal, and medical judgment that resuscitation would be inappropriate because it "could do no good."[20]

The 1992 National Conference on Cardiopulmonary Resuscitation (CPR) and Emergency Cardiac Care (ECC) advanced the discussion by addressing even more explicitly the question of physician unilateral decision making on the basis of futility:

In certain circumstances CPR can be predicted to be unsuccessful and may be considered futile. . . . Physicians should not be obligated to provide futile therapy when asked to do so by patients or surrogates. . . . Medical futility justifies unilateral decisions by physicians to withhold or terminate resuscitation under the following circumstances:

1. Appropriate basic life support (BLS) and advanced life support (ALS) have already been attempted without restoration of circulation or breathing.

2. No physiological benefit from BLS or ALS can be expected because a patient's vital functions are deteriorating despite maximum therapy.

3. No survivors after CPR have been reported under the given circumstances in well-designed studies, for example, . . . patients with metastatic cancer.

In these strictly defined situations, the decision to stop or withhold resuscitation is appropriately a medical judgment. Patients should be informed of the no-CPR order but not offered the choice of CPR.[21]

Under the circumstances of what the guidelines call "strict" futility, the fact of futility is sufficient to justify physician unilateral decision making. The guidelines then go on to distinguish between "strict" futility and what they identify as a "looser, less objective" kind of futility. Only the former would justify physician unilateral decision making. As an instance of a looser kind of futility judgment, the guidelines cite the case of a physician who regards CPR to be futile for a young patient in a persistent vegetative state. The guidelines explain that though CPR may not restore cerebral function, it might restore circulation and facilitate long-term survival. Therefore, the physician would be making a value judgment about which goals are worth pursuing. The guidelines' other example of a looser kind of futility judgment involves a physician who regards CPR to be futile because the reported survival rate after CPR is low, but not zero percent. Again, the guidelines explain that the physician would be making a value judgment, this time about what probability of success is worthwhile. In each example, the physician would be unwarranted in imposing her value judgment on the patient. Unilaterally deciding not to attempt resuscitation on the basis of a factual futility judgment is described as justified and appropriate, while doing the same on the basis of an evaluative futility judgment is characterized as inappropriate.

In the 1989 second edition of its *Ethics Manual*, the American College of Physicians similarly considered who should ultimately be empowered to make decisions about resuscitation.

The two guiding principles that should determine whether a DNR order is written for a competent patient are the medical indications and the patient's preferences.

When treatment is judged useless, or when CPR would only prolong the dying process, then, if the patient agrees with the plan, an order not to resuscitate such a patient is ethical. In cases of conflict between the competent patient and the physician, the patient's wishes should prevail. For reasons of conscience, the physician may elect to withdraw from the case. . . .

[For patients who lack decision making capacity,] even when resuscitation would provide no medical benefit, the family should be told the medical situation, and the physician should attempt to persuade them of the reasonableness of a DNR order.[22]

Three years later, in the third edition of its *Ethics Manual*, the American College of Physicians took up more directly the question of the options available to a physician when discussion and persuasion fail and a patient continues to insist on resuscitation deemed futile by the physician.

The physician should make every effort to ensure that misunderstanding, poor communication, or unaddressed psychosocial concerns are not the reasons for an apparently irrational insistence on resuscitation. [Then,] if physicians write a unilateral DNR order, they must inform the patient.[23]

Underlying all of these position statements is the belief that physicians should judge the appropriateness or inappropriateness of CPR apart from patient preferences. Behind medical judgments of inappropriateness are the dual concerns that resuscitation sometimes would not work and sometimes would not be worth it. These concerns have surfaced in the growing body of literature as attempts are made to identify the kinds of patients for whom, and the kinds of medical conditions for which, CPR either would not work or would not be worth it. Because arguments are often made using futility as the common currency, the ongoing discussion about appropriate resuscitation remains important to the futility debate.

Other medical specialties have also entered the discussion and produced position statements that have broadened the dialogue on futility. A consensus panel of the American College of Chest Physicians and the Society of Critical Care Medicine (ACCP/SCCM) offered its "Ethical and Moral Guidelines for the Initiation, Continuation, and Withdrawal of Intensive Care" in 1990. Though they recognize the importance of involving patients and their surrogates in the selection of therapeutic goals and subsequent decision making, the guidelines also endorse in certain circumstances the legitimacy of unilateral decisions based on medical judgments of futility.

> Sometimes patients without decision making capacity are assessed by the physiologic futility standard—ie, no treatment is available that can achieve any medical goals. . . . [In such cases, though] ambiguous, [the] concept of futility can be used to justify unilateral decisions by physicians to withhold or withdraw life-sustaining treatment. [To summarize the decision making framework applicable to all patients,] therapy is defined as those interventions which can be reasonably expected to benefit the patient. . . . If general medical opinion considers a particular treatment futile (not altering the patient's immediate survival nor offering any advantage over alternative treatments), then this alternative need not be performed or even discussed with the patient and/or his surrogate.[24]

While the recommendations are qualified slightly if "statistical likelihood of survival or improvement is as low as 5 percent,"[25] futility is promoted as a viable concept for physician driven ethical decision making.

A similar approach is taken by the American Thoracic Society in their 1991 official statement on "Withholding and Withdrawing Life-Sustaining Therapy." Taking as its purpose the defining of acceptable standards of medical practice, the statement includes a section on limiting life sustaining medical interventions without patient or surrogate consent when the intervention is judged to be futile.

> The purpose of a life-sustaining intervention should be to restore or maintain a patient's well-being; and it should not have as its sole goal the unqualified prolongation of a patient's biological life. On this basis, a life-sustaining intervention may be withheld or withdrawn from a patient without the consent of the patient or surrogate if the intervention is judged to be futile. A life-sustaining intervention is futile if reasoning and experience indicate that the intervention would be highly unlikely to result in a meaningful survival for that patient.[26]

Following this increasingly popular approach, the American Medical Association's Council on Ethical and Judicial Affairs offered its "Guidelines for the Appropriate Use of Do-Not-Resuscitate Orders" in 1991:

> A physician is not ethically obligated to make a specific diagnostic or therapeutic procedure available to a patient, even on specific request, if the use of such a procedure would be futile. . . . In the unusual circumstance when efforts to resuscitate a patient are judged by the treating physician to be futile, *even if previously requested by the patient*, CPR may be withheld.[27]

In its 1994 *Code of Medical Ethics*, the American Medical Association's Council on Ethical and Judicial Affairs affirmed that physicians are not obligated to provide treatment demanded by patients, and that patient consent is not necessary for a physician to forego resuscitation attempts.

> If, in the judgment of the attending physician, it would be inappropriate to pursue CPR, the attending physician may enter a do-not-resuscitate order into the patient's record.[28]

The Council eschews the concept of futility "which cannot be meaningfully defined,"[29] in favor of the association's general Principles of Medical Ethics and Council Opinion Statements. Consistent with the general approach taken by other professional societies, the Council submits,

> Physicians are not ethically obligated to deliver care that, in their best professional judgment, will not have a reasonable chance of benefitting their patients.[30]

Taken together, these professional position statements offer substantial support to practitioners who want to unilaterally refuse to provide treatment. While these statements rarely offer an analysis or defense of their preferred definition and use of futility or related concepts, they have nonetheless been influential in shaping and advancing the futility discussion.

Institutional or Community Policies

Along with the growing number of position statements that appeal to futility as a ground for unilateral refusal to provide treatment, the Joint Commission of Accreditation of Healthcare Organizations (JCAHO) requirements for institutional policies on issues ranging from brain death to DNR orders, to withholding and withdrawing life support, have further expanded the health care professional's awareness of the concept of futility and its potential applications. Since hospital policies must usually specify the conditions under which treatments may be foregone and the steps that must be taken before treatments are withdrawn, they typically include discussions of the concept of futility, however incomplete or problematic.

Interest in taking a more direct proactive stand on the problem of futility and in granting physicians authority to make unilateral decisions based on futility has also grown. Increasingly, institutions are experimenting with the use of explicit futility policies, and groups of hospitals are contemplating the adoption of community or regional futility policies that would specify in advance treatments that would be considered futile and would therefore not be provided.[31] The proposals take a variety of forms.

The Santa Monica Hospital Medical Center's Futile Care Guidelines have received wide publicity. Reprinted in several national publications,[32] the guidelines address situations in which the attending physician deems further treatment to be futile, but the patient or the patient's family insists on continuing treatment. The policy defines futile care as:

> Any clinical circumstance in which the doctor and his consultants, consistent with the available medical literature, conclude that further treatment (except comfort care) cannot, within a reasonable possibility, cure, ameliorate, improve, or restore a quality of life that would be satisfactory to the patient.

As examples of futile care they list:

1. Irreversible coma or persistent vegetative state
2. Terminally ill and the application of life sustaining procedure would serve only to artificially delay the moment of death
3. Permanent dependence on ICU care

The guidelines specify that if all the prescribed steps are taken and the patient or the patient's family remain unconvinced, "neither the doctor nor the hospital is required to provide care that is not medically indicated." The guidelines leave open the option of transferring care of the patient to another physician and/or hospital.

Johns Hopkins Hospital in Baltimore takes a similar approach in its policy on withholding and withdrawing futile life saving interventions:

> Any course of treatment may be regarded as futile if it is highly unlikely to have a beneficial outcome, or if it is highly likely merely to preserve permanent unconsciousness or persistent vegetative state or require permanent hospitalization in an intensive care unit. . . . It is the policy of [this hospital] that attending physicians are not required to offer life sustaining intervention, and may refuse a request for the same, if the intervention is medically futile and will not offer meaningful benefit to the patient. . . . [If a conflict arises and persists,] the attending physician or the patient may seek an alternative attending physician.[33]

Some hospitals in the same region have considered taking a more stringent stand, prohibiting the provision of futile care by any physician or institution within a specified geographic area. For example, California's San Bernardino County Medical Society initially proposed and later rejected[34] guidelines that would allow physicians to terminate treatment they deemed medically inappropriate or futile once the physician, a second medical opinion, and the institution's bioethics committee were all in agreement that the treatment was futile. An early draft of the guidelines included a novel provision that precluded transfer to another physician or hospital within the area for receipt of treatment deemed futile in accordance with the guidelines. This clause, addressing the tendency of patients to "physician shop," was eliminated in later drafts of the proposal.

A different approach is being tried in Denver with the GUIDe Project (Guidelines for the Use of Intensive Care in Denver.)[35] The intention of the project, which began in April 1993, is to forge consensus about futility within and between the health care community and the lay population. What distinguishes this approach is the project's steadfast and careful commitment to using an inclusive long-term process for consensus building. Subcommittees (adult intensive care, neonatal intensive care, and long term care) have been meeting regularly and attempting to achieve their own consensus on proposals that are then presented at plenary sessions. Based on feedback received at the plenary sessions, proposals are revised and resubmitted. As proposals develop, they are subject to continuous review by health professionals and the general public. The expectation is that area-wide futility guidelines will be developed out of this extended process of consensus building.

Other efforts have focussed on the development of procedural, rather than substantive, guidelines that multiple institutions in a common geographic area could support. In 1995, for example, a multi-institution task force on medical futility drawn from a wide range of institutions in the greater Houston area met and ultimately produced "Guidelines on Institutional Policies on the Determination of Medically Inappropriate Interventions."[36] The policy offers a conflict resolution mechanism for cases in which patients demand treatment deemed medically inappropriate by the responsible physician. Recommended procedures include full disclosure by the physician to the patient whenever the physician judges a desired treatment to be futile, the option to transfer care, the receipt of a second medical opinion, and the use of an institutional review process for persistent conflicts. The policy stipulates that the institutional review body's agreement is necessary for a physician to withhold or withdraw treatment deemed medically inappropriate. Once that determination has been made and supported, transfer to another physician to provide the intervention in question is not allowed.

Curiously, while the Houston policy provides for patient participation, and explicitly rejects physician unilateral decision making, the recommended process relies on an exclusively physician driven and institutionally grounded approach. In fact, the policy was developed without either meaningful or substantial participation of the lay public (a shortcoming acknowledged by the organizers of the effort), and the recommended procedures provide no particular protection for patients whose values might be in conflict with the physicians and institutions reviewing their requests.

Some would argue, nonetheless, that thoughtful institutional futility policies provide a far more defensible warrant for decision making than decisions driven primarily by individual physicians or individual patients. Tom L. Tomlinson and Diane Czlonka contend that the prospective development of such policies can assist physicians in avoiding some of the most common traps in futility conflicts. Focussing specifically on the case of futile resuscitation, they argue that hospital policies requiring patient consent for DNR orders are fundamentally misguided since they encourage contemplation of "bogus choices." They favor instead the development of hospital futility policies that would specifically grant physicians authority to make decisions consistent with the recognized values of their profession.

While recognizing practical problems in their implementation, Tomlinson and Czlonka suggest that such policies can be part of the solution since they offer a new context for the necessary conversation between physicians and patients:

> Adamant demands for futile resuscitation are less likely when the goal of discussion is not to have the patient make a choice, but rather to gain their understanding and acceptance of the choice already made and presented by the physician against attempting resuscitation.[37]

This approach highlights the importance of developing consensus between the medical profession and the public about the kinds of decisions physicians ought to be authorized to make. I take up the matter more fully in Chapter 5. For now it is sufficient to note that most futility policies fail to address adequately the genuine disagreement between the medical profession and the lay population over the definition and assessment of beneficial treatment and the appropriate scope of physician authority. A recent consensus statement of the Society of Critical Care Medicine stands as a notable exception in this regard, recommending that policies limiting treatment "reflect moral values acceptable to the community."[38]

In the end, despite the popularity of institutional or community based futility policies, significant questions remain concerning both their ultimate legitimacy and their potential for successfully adjudicating intractable futility conflicts.

Case Law and Statutes

The legal system is the final arena in which the discussion of futility has emerged in a preliminary form. Though there has yet to be a definitive case or statutory answer to the problem of futility, the legal system has certainly had a role in stimulating and advancing the discussion.

Probably the most influential court ruling was the 1983 case of Mr. Clarence Herbert, though the ruling never answered explicitly the question of whether physician unilateral decision making on the grounds of futility was legally permissible. After undergoing routine surgery for closure of an ileostomy, Mr. Herbert had an unexpected cardiorespiratory arrest in the recovery room, leading to a diagnosis of permanent brain damage with permanent vegetative state likely. At his family's request, three days after the arrest, the physicians discontinued Mr. Herbert's ventilatory support. Two days later, his intravenously supplied nutrition and hydration were withdrawn. Responding to a nurse's concerns, the district attorney charged Mr. Herbert's physicians, Drs. Nejdl and Barber, with murder in the first degree and conspiracy to commit murder.

The California Appellate Court dropped the charges against the two physicians and offered a preliminary legal response to the question of futility. After establishing that the physicians' actions did not constitute homicide under California law, the court went on to explain that physicians have no duty to provide ineffective treatment, or treatment that provides no benefit.

> A physician has no duty to continue treatment, once it has proved to be ineffective. Although there may be a duty to provide life-sustaining machinery in the *immediate* aftermath of a cardio-respiratory arrest, there is no duty to continue its use once it has become futile in the opinion of qualified medical personnel. . . . [Citing a President's Commission source, the opinion continues,] A physician is authorized under the standards of medical practice to discontinue a form of therapy which in his medical judgment is useless. . . . By useless is meant that the continued use of the therapy cannot and does not improve the prognosis for recovery.[39]

Recognizing that these comments provide little guidance for determining that further treatment will be of no reasonable benefit to the patient, for deciding when such a determination should be made, or for resolving conflicts over the determination, the court deliberately refers these questions to the legislature and the medical community for more thorough consideration and resolution.

It is important to realize that it would be contrary to the court's stated intent to rely on *Barber* as an answer to the problem of futility and to cite it as a justification for unilateral refusal to provide treatment. Furthermore, it is inconsistent with the facts of the case to use *Barber* to justify physician unilateral refusal to provide requested treatment against the express wishes of patients. In contrast to the paradigmatic futility case in which physicians want to deny treatment that they unilaterally deem futile, despite patient preference and often without their involvement, Mr. Herbert's family concurred with his physicians' assessment. In fact, their agreement was the driving force behind the decision to discontinue support.

Another case frequently cited to support physician refusal of requested treatment is the 1990 case of Baby L.[40] This case involved a two-year-old patient diagnosed in utero with fetal hydronephrosis and oligohydramnios, delivered at 36 weeks with respiratory distress, and treated over the course of the next two years for recurrent pneumonias, sepsis, and cardiopulmonary arrests. Given her neurologic damage and poor prognosis, the patient's physicians, contrary to her mother's wishes, judged further intervention not to be in her best interest. When the physicians voiced their unwillingness to continue aggressive treatment, the mother brought the issue to probate court. Though the legal question was rendered moot when a consulting pediatric neurologist agreed to take over the case, and though the court never answered the question of whether physicians could be forced to provide care that they deemed contrary to the best interest of their patient, the *Baby L* case may have set the stage for future cases of physician refusal, on the grounds of futility, to provide requested treatment.

Since neither *Barber* nor *Baby L* provided definitive answers to the question of how physicians should respond in the face of requests for treatments that they deem futile, expectations for a forthcoming answer were only heightened and then dashed with the 1991 *Wanglie* case.[41] Mrs. Helga Wanglie, an 87-year-old woman with preexisting lung disease, was admitted to Hennepin County Hospital with pneumonia following a hip fracture. Once stabilized, though still ventilator-dependent, she was transferred to a long-term care facility. Following a cardiac arrest during an unsuccessful attempt to wean her from the ventilator, Mrs. Wanglie was transferred back to Hennepin County Hospital. There her family agreed not to contest a DNR order, but refused to authorize discontinuation of ventilatory support, even in the face of the diagnosis that she was in a persistent vegetative state. Though careful not to use the word futility to support their position, the physicians at Hennepin County Hospital argued that continued treatment was not in Mrs. Wanglie's personal medical interest and requested judicial backing for their refusal to provide it.

At issue again was whether physicians could refuse to provide requested treatment based on their judgments of the treatment's effectiveness and desirability. And again, the courts failed to give a definitive legal answer. Responding only to the narrow question with which they had been presented, that is, whether Mr. Wanglie was the appropriate guardian and spokesperson for Mrs. Wanglie, the court confirmed that Mr. Wanglie was the appropriate guardian without explicitly affirming his decision to continue use of the ventilator. Thus the court successfully dodged the most delicate questions in the case.

Another important case is that of Stephanie Herrell, or Baby K,[42] as she was known in the court record and news coverage of the case. Stephanie was diagnosed in utero as anencephalic. Her mother refused the recommended abortion and insisted, on religious grounds, that she would carry her baby to term. Stephanie was delivered by c-section and was aggressively resuscitated at birth in accordance with her mother's wishes.

Shortly after her birth, Stephanie's physicians tried to convince her mother to agree to a DNR order and to permit discontinuation of ventilatory support, explaining that there was no treatment for anencephaly and that further treatment was unnecessary and inappropriate. When Stephanie's mother refused, the physicians consulted the hospital's ethics committee. A subcommittee of the ethics committee (composed of a family practitioner, a psychiatrist, and a minister) reviewed the case and concluded that ventilatory support was futile and should be discontinued. The committee recommended that if the mother still refused, the case should be referred to the legal system for review.

When she was almost six weeks old, Stephanie was transferred to a nursing home at a time when she was not in respiratory distress and was therefore not in need of ventilatory support. The transfer was made on the condition that the hospital take her back again if she required ventilatory support, a treatment not available at the nursing home. Several times in the following few months, Stephanie was readmitted to the hospital in respiratory distress. Each time she was eventually stabilized, weaned from the ventilator, and transferred back to the nursing home.

Stephanie's mother visited her regularly and remained firm in her belief that God would work a miracle if that was his will. Otherwise, as was later described in the court opinion, she believed that God, and not other humans, should decide the moment of her daughter's death. The hospital, Stephanie's physicians, her biological father (reported to be otherwise uninvolved), and an appointed guardian ad litem all disagreed with Stephanie's mother and argued that ventilatory treatment should be withheld the next time Stephanie developed respiratory distress.

The hospital finally brought the case to district court for a declaratory judgment. The court ruled that there was in fact an obligation to provide the treatment in question, based on the Emergency Medical Treatment and Active Labor (EMTALA) law, the Rehabilitation Act of 1973, and the Americans with Disabilities Act. The court located further support for its opinion in the 14th Amendment's due process clause, which they interpreted as giving parents the right to bring their children up as they saw fit, the 1st Amendment's freedom of religion clause, the presumption of a natural bond of affection between parents and children that makes parents the most appropriate decision makers, and the general presumption in favor of life, all else being equal.

Much to the surprise of the medical community, the appellate court upheld the district court's decision, grounding their decision in the EMTALA law alone. In other words, the hospital had a duty to admit and stabilize Stephanie whenever she presented in respiratory distress. The U.S. Supreme Court later declined to hear the case.

I discuss the *Baby K* case further in Chapter 4, with respect to the problem of medical uncertainty and mistakes. For now, it is enough to note that while the *Baby K* case ultimately was decided in favor of the mother, the problem of whether physicians can unilaterally refuse to provide treatment on the basis of futility was never the explicit focus of the courts' attention. In that respect, the *Baby K* decision is a narrow one because, like the *Barber*, *Baby L*, and *Wanglie* decisions, it does not provide a direct legal ruling on the concept of medical futility. The appellate court decision clearly states:

> It is beyond the limits of our judicial function to address the moral or ethical propriety of providing emergency stabilizing medical treatment to anencephalic infants. Congress . . . required hospitals and physicians to

provide stabilizing care to any individual presenting in an emergency medical condition. EMTALA does not carve out an exception for anencephalic infants in respiratory distress any more than it carves out an exception for comatose patients, those with lung cancer, or those with muscular dystrophy—all of whom may repeatedly seek emergency stabilizing treatment for respiratory distress and also possess an underlying medical condition that severely affects their quality of life and ultimately may result in their death.[43]

Again, the court advised, if Congress wishes to make a different determination, it is free to reexamine and revise existing laws.

The most recent futility case to reach the court system at this writing involves Catherine Gilgunn, a patient hospitalized at Massachusetts General Hospital. In 1995 a jury ruled that Massachusetts General and two of its physicians were not guilty of neglect or imposing emotional distress when they acted against Mrs. Gilgunn's acknowledged wishes to sustain her life.[44] Mrs. Gilgunn was a 71-year-old woman with a prior history of diabetes, heart disease, Parkinson's disease, chronic urinary tract infections, breast cancer, a stroke, and three hip replacements. Prior to a fourth hip replacement, she suffered a series of repeated and uncontrollable seizures that caused irreversible brain damage and left Mrs. Gilgunn in a coma, on life support in the intensive care unit at Massachusetts General. Her physicians, with the concurrence of the "optimum care committee," recommended a DNR order. Mrs. Gilgunn's daughter objected, claiming that her mother had always wanted every available medical procedure done to keep her alive as long as possible, and insisting that her mother's wishes be honored. Ultimately a DNR order was written, allegedly without the daughter's knowledge. Mrs. Gilgunn allegedly was weaned from the ventilator and died shortly thereafter of respiratory distress.[45]

What distinguishes this case from the *Baby L, Wanglie,* and *Baby K* cases is that the physicians took proactive steps without first asking the courts for a declaratory judgment that they would not be in violation of any laws for refusing to provide the treatment deemed futile. What further differentiates the case is that for the first time a jury was asked to deliberate explicitly on the issue of medical futility. In response to the question of whether Mrs. Gilgunn would have wanted to receive CPR or to be kept on a ventilator if she had been able to express herself, the jury answered yes. In response to the question of whether such treatment was futile, the jury again answered yes. Open to question, of course, are the nature and scope of the instructions given to the jury with respect to the definition of futility and the extent of physicians' obligations to provide or not to provide futile treatment. While provocative, the *Gilgunn* decision has no precedential weight since the trial court's verdict was never appealed.[46]

In light of the above cases, we must note that though the courts have come close to pronouncing judgment on the problem of futility, they have yet to provide clear and definitive guidance about the legal status of physician unilateral decision making on the basis of futility.

With the exception of the 1985 Federal Child Abuse Amendments enacted in response to the Baby Doe controversy in the early 1980s, the government has also rarely addressed directly the issue of whether physicians might be permitted to forego treatment they deem futile. Under the Child Abuse Amendments, in order to qualify for federal funds, state child protection agencies must have in place a mechanism for responding to reports of medical neglect, including the withholding of medically indicated treatment from disabled infants with life threatening conditions. The amendments define the following as exceptions to the requirement that all medically indicated treatment, including appropriate nutrition, hydration, and medication, be provided:

> The infant is chronically and irreversibly comatose; or the provision of such treatment would merely prolong dying or not be effective in ameliorating or correcting all of the infant's life-threatening conditions, or otherwise be futile in terms of the survival of the infant; or the provision of such treatment would be virtually futile in terms of the survival of the infant and the treatment itself under such circumstances would be inhumane.[47]

Citing "futile in terms of survival" or "virtually futile" as exceptions further solidified the use of futility in medical decision making, but did little to clarify the ultimate questions raised by futility judgments in the first place.

Various state legislatures have similarly attempted to include futility as an exception in their statutes governing the provision, withholding, or withdrawing of treatments ranging from CPR to other life sustaining interventions.[48] But like the Child Abuse Amendments, they offer little in the way of clarification or argumentation regarding the appropriate meaning and use of appeals to futility.

In fact, though explicit references and preliminary responses to the problem of futility can be found in established guidelines, professional position statements, institutional policies, and case and statutory law, the discussion to date has not resolved definitively the question of whether futility is a sufficient justification for physician unilateral refusal to offer, provide, or continue treatment.

Factors Leading to the Current Futility Debate

Because the proposal of physician unilateral decision making differs so starkly from the response to medical limitation made only a few decades ago, it is helpful to step back and trace the factors that might have led to this development.

An earlier answer to the question of end-of-life decision making in the clinical context, which now seems to have fallen out of favor, was offered by Sharon H. Imbus and Bruce E. Zawacki in their 1977 article, "Autonomy for Burned Patients When Survival Is Unprecedented."[49] According to Imbus and Zawacki, it is precisely at the moment when further medical intervention is recognized by all to be futile with respect to survival, when there is "nothing more that medical science can offer," that the decision (about whether to proceed on an aggressive course, or to opt instead for comfort measures only) is turned over to the patient. A medical judgment of futility is offered so that patients can factor it into their decision about how to proceed; but the medical judgment that limitation has been reached does not itself become the decision.

Even when survival is statistically unprecedented, or, in today's jargon, when treatment is futile from a medical perspective, Imbus and Zawacki continue to place the highest value on the capacity and right of autonomous agents to determine what happens to their bodies and to choose their treatment course.

As the growing body of literature on futility attests, the predominant position today runs completely contrary to the Imbus-Zawacki model. Many health care professionals argue that it is precisely at the moment when further medical intervention is recognized to be futile, when limitation has been reached, when there is "nothing more that medical science can offer," that the decision becomes a medical one and is taken away from the patient. Accordingly, foregoing or continuing treatment becomes exclusively physician rather than patient directed.

A number of factors have contributed to this shift in paradigm case and response to futility. First, changes in the conceptual framework used to evaluate treatment options has influenced the language and line of argumentation. Second, changes in the understanding of the nature of the question have led to a reevaluation of the distribution of power, authority, and expertise. Third, closer consideration of the actual nature and scope of the principle of autonomy has led to questions about the patient's appropriate role in medical decision making. Fourth, concerns about the just allocation of scarce health care resources have led to an increased perception of the need to set limits. Together, these four factors explain the context in which the futility debate has arisen. In order to provide a broad sense of that context, I will examine each factor in turn.

Changes in the Conceptual Framework for Evaluating Treatment Options

The source of a key conceptual issue in the futility debate can be traced to the shift away from a focus on whether a particular treatment is ordinary (and therefore obligatory) or extraordinary (and therefore supererogatory) to the now preferred focus on proportionality, that is, on whether the attendant burdens of a particular treatment are proportionate to its anticipated benefits and usefulness.

While considerable attention has been devoted to the meaning and appropriate application of the proportionality test, only recently in the futility debate has the moral meaning and weight of one component of that test—usefulness or uselessness—become the subject of equally critical discussion.

In its report *Deciding to Forego Life-Sustaining Treatment*, the President's Commission for the Study of Ethical Problems in Medicine and Biomedical and Behavioral Research closely followed developments in Catholic moral theology by rejecting the ordinary/extraordinary distinction in favor of the proportionality test. The Commission identified and rejected two of the most popular meanings ascribed to the ordinary/extraordinary distinction: the statistical and the technological.[50] According to the statistical interpretation of the distinction, standard, customary, or usual treatments are ordinary; unusual, uncommon, rarely done treatments are extraordinary. Under the technological interpretation, simple, easily done treatments are ordinary; complex, elaborate, or artificial treatments are extraordinary. Noting that neither interpretation distinguished treatments on sufficiently morally relevant grounds, the Commission rejected them both in favor of an interpretation developed by Catholic theologians.

In adopting the theological interpretation, the President's Commission was not endorsing or subscribing to the overall teachings of Catholic moral theology, but rather recognizing and appreciating its direct applications to controversies in bioethics. In fact, Catholic theologians had already explicitly been considering under what circumstances, if any, it would be morally acceptable to withhold or withdraw life sustaining technology. In an attempt to delineate the scope of patient and physician obligation, early answers to the question distinguished treatments that were morally required from treatments that were morally optional. Under this construct, ordinary treatments were deemed obligatory for patients to accept and for others to provide, while extraordinary treatments were deemed supererogatory for patients to accept and for others to provide. Rather than appraising a treatment's technological or statistical ordinariness or extraordinariness, moral theologians focussed instead on a given treatment's usefulness and burdensomeness in the context of a particular patient's life. The President's Commission found this shift in perspective helpful.

In 1958, Pope Pius XII articulated the position of the Catholic church when he explained the distinction between ordinary and extraordinary treatment and its import for the general duty to preserve life and health. The duty is simply a duty

> to use only ordinary means—according to circumstances of persons, places, times and culture—that is, those that do not involve any grave burden for oneself or another. . . . [When] treatment [goes] beyond the ordinary means to which one is bound, it cannot be held that there is an obligation to use them nor, consequently, that one is bound to give the doctor permission to use them.[51]

This statement yielded several insights. First, it refined the distinction between ordinary and extraordinary treatments and the different obligations individuals have to employ them. Second, and importantly for the contemporary futility debate, it presumed a specific relationship between patients and their physicians. The Pope clearly states,

> The rights and duties of the doctor are correlative to those of the patient. The doctor, in fact, has no separate or independent right where the patient is concerned.[52]

One could conclude that the Pope's language implies the appropriateness of subsuming physician rights and duties under patient rights and duties. Under this model, patients make the initial judgment about whether they are permitted lawfully and obligated morally to use particular interventions and, consequently and secondarily, whether they will grant the physician permission to use them. A physician's obligations correlate with her patient's moral obligations, not with an abstract sense of medicine's traditional goals or of the integrity of the profession. This insight poses a direct challenge to the current approach advocated by futility proponents. Similarly, this early work calls our attention to the fact that treatment options can be evaluated from either an objective or subjective stance, and that an appropriate perspective must be chosen. For the Pope, benefits and burdens must be judged from the individual patient's perspective and not from a removed objective stance.[53]

In 1980, the Vatican *Declaration on Euthanasia* offered refinements to the question of what circumstances, if any, render morally acceptable the withholding or withdrawing of life sustaining technology. This time the Vatican asked, "Is it necessary in all circumstances to have recourse to all possible remedies?"[54] Recognizing the problematic features of the ordinary/extraordinary distinction, the Vatican's answer began by recommending a conceptual and linguistic shift away from the ordinary/extraordinary distinction in favor of the concept of proportionality. Under this new construct, when the burdens of a given treatment are disproportionate to its benefits and usefulness, it may be foregone. The President's Commission and the secular bioethics community similarly followed this conceptual and linguistic shift.

While calling for the shift, the Vatican Declaration also raised new questions about the appropriate relationship between physicians and patients. While the Declaration did not address explicitly the question of how to resolve conflicts that might arise in assessing whether a treatment's benefits, usefulness, and burdens are proportionate or disproportionate, it seemed to place less emphasis[55] on the primacy of the patient's determination than either Pope Pius XII or the President's Commission.

In fact, while the Vatican Declaration specified factors that might be considered in assessing whether a particular treatment constitutes a proportionate or disproportionate means of prolonging life, and though it acknowledged the relevance of patient consent and family wishes, it characterized physicians as more expert in making the critical assessments. In reference to patient recourse to the most advanced or even experimental and risky medical techniques, and to the interruption of their use once begun, the Vatican explained:

> It is also permitted, with the patient's consent, to interrupt these means, where the results fall short of expectations. But for such a decision to be made, account will have to be taken of the reasonable wishes of the patient's family, as also of the advice of the *doctors* who *are specially competent* in the matter. The latter *may in particular judge that the investment in instruments and personnel is disproportionate to the results foreseen; they may also judge that the techniques applied impose on the patient strain or suffering out of proportion with the benefits which he or she may gain from such techniques.*[56]

According to this reading, doctors, and not patients or family members, are best qualified to judge whether treatments are worth pursuing. Doctors, and not patients or family members, are best qualified to judge whether the strain or suffering a patient may endure are proportionate to the benefits she might receive. And finally, doctors are given the latitude to weigh equally the effects of investing in instruments and personnel with the effects treatments might have on patients. What is not clear is whether doctors can withhold or withdraw treatments they have judged to be disproportionate means to prolong life if they cannot gain patient consent. This quandary is now at the heart of the contemporary futility debate.

Three key questions are at issue in this body of literature and the contemporary futility debate that grew, in part, out of it. First, how (according to what criteria) should treatments be assessed? Second, who is best qualified to make judgments about a treatment's desirability and appropriateness? Third, what decisions and actions should follow, once a judgment has been made?

As proportionality replaced the ordinary/extraordinary distinction first in theological and then in secular scholarly thought, these questions became even more complex. By what and whose criteria should a treatment's burdens be judged proportionate or disproportionate to its benefits and usefulness? Are there universally accepted definitions of benefit, burden, and usefulness? If a treatment is gravely burdensome does that mean that it is useless? How should conflicts over judgments of proportionality be resolved? Clearly these are the questions that must be, but have not yet been, addressed seriously and directly by futility proponents.

Changes in the Physician-Patient Relationship

The second factor contributing to the shift in paradigm case and re-sponse to limitation in the futility debate is the changing understanding of the nature of the physician-patient relationship and the distribution of power, authority, and expertise. At issue is the appropriate nature of the therapeutic relationship between physicians and their patients, and behind the various arguments represented in the futility literature are radically dif-ferent visions of the shape that this relationship should take.

When bioethics began to address the question of appropriate treatment decision making at the end of life, it became clear that the question of whether to withhold or withdraw life sustaining treatment could not be an-swered conclusively from an exclusively medical or scientific perspective. Modern technology had introduced a new level of choices to which medi-cine could not claim to have exclusive answers, because the answers turned on questions of values and not just on questions of science. For example, would terminally ill patients prefer to live longer or suffer less? If the choice were between continued biological existence and existence only at a certain quality of life, which would be selected? Obviously, unless they knew the patient's particular values and goals, physicians could not claim to know the answers to these questions. Because it offered no way of capturing or incor-porating the patient's value-rich answer to the question of whether a par-ticular treatment was desirable or appropriate, the historical precedent of physician dominated decision making with little or no patient involvement was revealed to be seriously lacking.

In fact, it was soon argued that no assessments of benefits, burdens, use-fulness, or uselessness could be strictly technical and objective; they all have an undeniable evaluative component. The obvious question became: who was in the best position to make an evaluative judgment about treatment options? Robert M. Veatch coined the phrase "generalization of expertise" to explain that it was no longer possible or justifiable for physicians to gen-eralize from one area of expertise—what medically and scientifically is the case—to another area of expertise—what normatively should be the case.[57] Because technical expertise cannot be generalized to evaluative expertise, physicians cannot claim exclusive competence to make unilateral judgments and decisions.[58]

Application of the generalization of expertise argument to the contem-porary dilemma suggests, for example, that while physicians may be more expert than others in assessing whether a particular patient is in a persistent vegetative state, that does not mean they are any more expert in assessing whether life in a persistent vegetative state is worth living, and therefore whether continued treatment is morally appropriate.

The persistent problem of deciding whose assessments, definitions, values, goals, and preferences should carry the most weight in the evolving relationship between physicians and patients has informed the contemporary futility debate. Should physicians be empowered to judge a particular treatment's desirability and appropriateness irrespective of patients's assessments, definitions, values, goals, and preferences? Or, if assessments are collaboratively made in the context of partnership rather than paternalism, are there still some interventions that should not be offered, continued, or provided despite patient requests? These are some of the questions at stake in the current futility debate.

A Reconsideration of the Nature and Scope of Patient Autonomy

The third way to understand the shift in paradigm case and response to limitation is to note the way in which the appropriate nature and scope of the principle of autonomy has been reconsidered in recent years. The older paradigm case of end-of-life decision making focussed on patients' negative rights, that is, the right to be left alone, the right to be free from unwanted interventions, and the right to refuse treatment.[59] Philosophically and legally, these rights were understood fundamentally to be rights of noninterference that derived from the basic rights to self-determination, privacy, and liberty.

In some respects the futility debate represents a response to the dramatic ascendency of the principle of respect for autonomy in the clinical context. As such, the futility debate serves as the occasion for reconsidering the actual meaning and limit of the concept of autonomy. Futility proponents have been quick to point to the problem of mistakenly blurring the distinction between the negative right of noninterference and the positive right of entitlement, and to the problem of elevating the principle of autonomy at the expense of other relevant moral appeals.

Many would argue that the principle of autonomy, understood as a principle of respect for persons, cannot be the basis for a right of access to treatment, whether "futile" or not. In other words, the acknowledgment of a patient's right to refuse a recommended treatment does not imply that patient's right to demand that a physician recommend or provide that same treatment. Those who extrapolate a right of access from a right to noninterference simply misunderstand the nature and scope of rights as well as the concept of respect for autonomy. Furthermore, other considerations, such as respect for professional integrity and commitments to beneficence and nonmaleficence, can constrain the autonomy-based rights patients would otherwise have.[60]

The challenge created by the current futility debate for those critical of the popular use of futility, then, is to identify any viable grounds other than autonomy that would be sufficient to compel a physician to provide treatment requested by the patient but deemed futile by the physician. I consider such alternative grounds to autonomy in Chapter 5.

Justice, Money, and the Allocation of Health Care Resources

A fourth and final factor that accounts for the dramatic shift in the clinical approach to so-called futile interventions merits discussion. To appreciate the full complexity of the futility debate, one must note the broader historical, economic, and political context in which it is situated. The context for the futility debate in this country has been one of dramatic change in the character and structure of the health care system. Physicians and patients grappling with medical decision making now do so in a climate characterized by a move away from traditional fee-for-service medicine in favor of systems of managed care, and in a context of complex and shifting incentives.[61] This restructuring has taken place in response to the perceived need to set limits and to reduce health care costs, a need increasingly acknowledged not only in the professional journals, but in the popular press as well.

And, as John D. Lantos points out, the shift in financial incentives caused by such restructuring has had a direct impact on the futility debate.

> Prior to prospective payment, doctors were apparently untroubled by patients' demands for "futile" treatments. Instead of arguing that it was unethical to provide such treatments, they generally argued that loyalty to their patients required that every potentially beneficial treatment be offered, that one couldn't put a price on life, that even if the chance of success was only one in a million, doctors would still be ethically obligated to provide it. When reimbursement incentives changed, so that doctors began to lose money instead of making money from providing such treatments, doctors suddenly discovered an ancient ethical obligation to refrain from providing such treatments.[62]

Though financial incentives are clearly not the only considerations that motivate physicians who appeal to futility as a justification for denying treatment, they have undeniably created a climate in which a treatment's so-called futility is more apt to be contemplated.

Concerns about justice and the allocation of scarce communal health care resources, and persistent calls for health care reform have also fueled the debate about futility. It is tempting to see our focus on futility as part of the solution to these concerns, since it would be irrational to spend our resources on treatment that all would deem futile. But, as I will show, appeals to futility are both shortsighted and misplaced in the context of the debate about scarce resources. They are shortsighted because there is no agreement on the meaning of futility or its relationship to cost-effectiveness, and so appeals to futility do little to advance the discussion. They are misplaced because concerns about futility and the just allocation of scarce resources are conceptually distinct, however related they may seem initially.

While attempts may be made to forego a particular treatment based on either consideration, concerns about futility and the just allocation of scarce resources are not necessarily related. Treatments foregone out of concern for their expense or scarce availability from the perspective of patient, family, provider, insurer, or society may or may not be futile. Similarly, treatments foregone out of concern for their futility from the perspective of patient, family, provider, insurer, or society may or may not be expensive or scarce. In other words, judgments about cost and just allocation do not necessarily correlate with judgments about futility. So while the current preoccupation with issues of scarcity and justice influences and perhaps even fuels the contemporary futility debate, it is important to distinguish the underlying concerns, and to note when they correspond and when they diverge.

In fact, the actual relationship between the futility debate and the growing concern about the just allocation of our scarce health care resources is far more complicated. Though concerns of futility and justice are, and should remain, conceptually distinct, concerns about cost are often the motivating force behind appeals to futility in the clinical setting, in the scholarly literature, and in the public policy arena. The concern is that we fairly allocate and spend our limited health care resources, which frequently means spending them on those treatment modalities and programs that have the greatest chance of benefitting the greatest number of deserving people.

From the perspective of these concerns, having the means to evaluate the likelihood of successful benefit and cost-effectiveness is absolutely essential. Evaluating the futility of particular interventions is one way of beginning to prioritize our efforts and rationalize our expenditure of limited resources. Additionally, having the means to make cost/benefit comparisons across patient and disease groups ensures that our collective resources are truly being used for the communal good.

Not surprisingly then, there is heightened interest in studying and documenting the actual effects of different medical interventions in a variety of patient populations in order to provide more clearly appropriate and cost-effective care. The outcomes movement is burgeoning and data bases are growing to meet the new demands. At the same time, scholars, practitioners, insurers, and policy makers alike are all exploring the applications of outcomes data to health care generally and to the problem of futility specifically.[63]

Ironically, the debate about whether patients have a right to treatment that their health care provider deems futile is taking place in a political climate that does not guarantee to all citizens either universal access to or a basic decent minimum of health care services. Philosophically, if there is not an acknowledged general right to health care, it would seem difficult to argue for a specific right to allegedly futile care.

But while this is a potential philosophical problem, in most futility cases, the patient has already gained at least minimal access to the health care system, and so the question raised is not typically one of access *per se*, but rather one of access to what the health care system potentially has to offer. Furthermore, even if we could ensure everyone universal access to a basic decent minimum, the futility problem would still persist. Patients might continue to insist on treatment deemed futile by their physicians. And physicians might still argue that they have a right to unilaterally refuse to provide treatment on the grounds of futility. So working to ensure adequate funding and access will not alone resolve the futility conflict.

In Chapter 5, I suggest that addressing questions of justice prospectively and democratically might help resolve some of the more difficult conflicts of futility that arise in the clinic and at the individual bedside. For now it is sufficient to note that concerns about justice and concerns about futility, while they may overlap in certain instances, are conceptually distinct.

Changes in the conceptual framework used to evaluate treatment options; changes in our understanding of the distribution of power, authority, and expertise in the physician-patient relationship; a reconsideration of the nature and scope of patient autonomy; and an increased concern about justice and the allocation of scarce health care resources have all influenced the development, nature, and scope of the contemporary futility debate. Together these factors help explain why futility has become such a contentious issue in the modern clinical setting, in the scholarly literature, and in the public policy arena. Their influence can be seen in the arguments represented on both sides of the futility debate.

The Nature of the Current Debate

The contemporary debate has been shaped by a core literature that has as its focus the appropriate meaning and use of futility judgments in the clinical setting. In the chapters that follow, I review critically the specific meanings and uses of futility put forth in the literature. For my purposes in this chapter, it suffices to characterize the broad nature of the arguments as they have appeared. The futility literature can be divided, at its most basic level, into contributions that argue in favor of and those that argue against appeals to futility as a sufficient justification for unilateral decision making in the clinical setting.

All of the key literature that argues in favor of appeals to futility in clinical judgment and decision making[64] seems to be motivated by a shared concern that acquiescing to patient demands for "futile" treatment will pervert the traditional goals of medicine (maximizing patient benefit while minimizing burden or risk of harm, preventing or curing disease, preventing or alleviating suffering, restoring function or health, et cetera) and undermine respect for professional autonomy and integrity (the ability and right of a professional to control the uses to which her knowledge and skill are put).

Though the specific contributions may differ in focus, emphasis, or presentation, the leading literature supporting appeals to futility follows a remarkably similar pattern of argumentation. Contributors rely substantially, though rarely explicitly, on the correlativity theory of rights and obligations. The implicit strategy is to so narrowly define and circumscribe the obligation of health care professionals, that the right of patients to receive "futile" treatment is eliminated.

Accordingly, the arguments typically begin with a presumption about the appropriate limits to obligatory and justified medical intervention. They generally assert, with little or no argument, that the only basis for the obligation to treat patients, and in fact the only justification for treatment comes from a commitment to the foundational principles of nonmaleficence and beneficence. From that assertion it follows easily that health care professionals are not obligated to provide, and in fact are not justified in providing, treatments that would be contrary to these principles. Next, the argument continues, providing "futile" treatment would be contrary to the principles of nonmaleficence and beneficence. The argument concludes, necessarily, that if health care professionals have no obligation to provide, then patients have no right to receive, "futile" treatment.

While this popular and familiar argument has gained prominence in the clinical setting, it is not immune to criticism in the literature. The key articles critical of appeals to futility in clinical judgment and decision making[65] all seem to be motivated by a concern that acquiescing to the current pressure to withhold or withdraw treatment on the grounds of futility, even against the express wishes of patients, will lead to inappropriate constraints on patient self determination, to regrettable sanctioning of health care professionals' already problematic tendency to generalize from one realm of expertise (e.g., what science or medicine can offer) to another (e.g., what is valuable, meaningful, and worth pursuing for patients), to an unfortunate return to an outdated form of paternalism, and to a violation of the contract between the medical profession and the lay population.

Again, though they may differ in focus, emphasis, or presentation, leading articles critical of appeals to futility follow a similar pattern of argumentation. In contrast to the argument that favors appeals to futility, the argument that criticizes such appeals generally considers respect for patient autonomy or fidelity, rather than adherence to the principles of nonmaleficence and beneficence, to be at the heart of the physician-patient encounter. Invading a patient's bodily integrity is not justified simply because the physician is technically competent and committed to the principles of nonmaleficence and beneficence. Such excursions into the patient's world are justified only when, and precisely because, the patient has consented to them. Further, presuming consensus between physician and patient regarding the meaning of harm that is to be avoided and benefit that is to be achieved, or regarding the traditional goals of medicine (or even the particular goals of a single medical encounter), begs the most important question. It is precisely because consensus on these definitions and goals has broken down and continues to break down between health care professionals and patients that futility and the right to control treatment decisions are such hotly contested problems in clinical practice.

With these objections in mind, those who argue against futility typically begin by asserting that all cases of futility are value-laden to varying degrees, though according to many, when it comes to justifying physician unilateral decision making, an exception can still legitimately be made of physiologic futility. The argument then claims that all treatment decisions involving value judgments properly belong to patients rather than to physicians. Next, it maintains that unilateral decision making by physicians is a form of unjustified paternalism (usually with the admission that there are some cases of justified paternalism, but that this is not one of them). The argument typically concludes that, with the exception of physiologically futile treatment, "futile" treatment cannot be unilaterally withheld or withdrawn. To do so would be an unjustified violation of patient autonomy, a regrettable slip into the generalization of expertise, an unwarranted act of paternalism, and a violation of the contract between the medical profession and the lay population.

Dividing the growing body of literature into these two fundamentally different approaches to the problem of futility is one helpful way of understanding the nature and scope of the contemporary futility debate. This book, however, goes beyond that descriptive level to consider the broad underlying assumptions that have shaped the current debate, to uncover the real issues at stake, and to point the way towards a more promising approach to conflicts over futility.

Because the fact/value distinction is widely accepted as the definitive philosophical analogue for judgments of futility, I have chosen to organize my critical evaluation of futility appeals around it. In Chapter 2 I offer a conceptual analysis of the concept of futility. Then, in Chapters 3 and 4 respectively, I consider whether futility appeals made on the grounds that treatment would be inappropriate, and futility appeals made on the grounds that treatment would be ineffective are, as currently formulated, sufficient to justify physician unilateral refusal to provide treatment. By demonstrating that neither formulation of futility is sufficient to justify physician unilateral refusals to provide treatment, I undercut the powerful appeal that the fact/value distinction holds in the contemporary futility debate. In Chapter 5 I extend my analysis and call for a reframing of the problem to better capture the moral appeals that are at the heart of seemingly intractable futility conflicts.

WHAT DO PEOPLE MEAN BY FUTILITY?
A Conceptual Analysis

WHILE THE PRACTICE of appealing to futility as a justification for withholding or withdrawing treatment has received increasing attention in the literature in the last decade, the concept of futility itself has yet to be the subject of a sufficiently systematic conceptual analysis. This chapter fills this gap in the existing discussion. Only after critical attention is given to the concept of futility itself can one thoroughly evaluate the normative arguments represented in the contemporary futility debate.

Though futility is referred to and appealed to extensively in the literature and the clinical setting, insufficient consideration has been given to two key epistemological questions raised by the concept. First, what is the definition or meaning of futility? Second, what are the acceptable criteria according to which futility can be recognized or known?

My conceptual analysis of futility will treat each epistemological question separately. To address the problem of identifying the appropriate definition and meaning of futility, I will consider the etymological roots of the word, as well as the meanings and definitions ascribed to the concept in the contemporary literature. To address the problem of selecting acceptable criteria according to which futile treatments could be recognized, I will consider procedural and substantive answers that have been offered in the contemporary discussion.

The Concept of Futility

The Etymological Roots

The Latin word *futilis* referred to actions or instruments which were inherently leaky and therefore ill-suited for achieving desired ends.[1] The implication was that the use of leaky means would always be in vain as the leak was an intrinsic defect that would make failure inevitable.

Recalling a relevant Greek myth, Schneiderman, Jecker, and Jonsen explain that

> The daughters of Danaus were condemned in Hades to draw water in leaky sieves, . . . [conveying, the authors suggest,] in all its fullness the meaning of the term [futility].[2]

According to the definition of *futilis*, despite their abilities, intentions, or desires, the daughters of Danaus were engaged in an inherently futile exercise. A related historical root of the term *futilis* refers to a religious vessel that, because of its awkward shape (wide at the top and narrow at the bottom) was impossible to fill without tipping over.[3]

Applying the notion of leakiness to medical interventions, one could infer that when failure to achieve a specified goal is inherent in a given treatment, the treatment can be defined as futile. Futile treatments are those that cannot achieve their prescribed goals, despite the abilities, intentions, or desires of those who employ them.

In terms of the Greek myth, futile medical interventions could be understood as leaky sieves or buckets. The bucket metaphor calls our attention to presumptions so ingrained in clinical education and practice that they are sometimes accepted as indisputable truths. The contemporary futility debate has been the occasion for exposing and calling into question the legitimacy of these long-accepted tenets of modern medicine.

Problems with the Leaky Bucket Metaphor

Though the leaky bucket metaphor and its underlying presumptions have been used, perhaps unwittingly, to support normative arguments in favor of physician authority to refuse unilaterally to provide treatment on the grounds of futility, neither the metaphor nor its underlying presumptions are problem-free.

First, an appeal to the leaky bucket metaphor to describe futile treatments presumes that there is consensus among clinicians and between clinicians and patients about what constitutes an effective and appropriate "bucket" for a given medical condition. As the contemporary futility debate attests, such consensus does not always exist.

In fact, the idea that a single treatment or set of treatments is effective and appropriate for a particular medical condition is simply not borne out by the historical legacy of modern medicine. The medical, biotechnological, and pharmaceutical industries all depend upon the fact that new treatments, as well as new applications for old treatments, are constantly the subject of scientific inquiry. Our understanding of effective and appropriate treatments is always evolving, and sometimes even changes dramatically.[4]

Similarly, the premise that a single treatment or set of treatments is effective and appropriate for a particular medical condition is inconsistent with the generally accepted notion of medicine as both an art and a science. As an art, medicine is practiced differently by different practitioners in different care settings in different times.

While a shared commitment to the scientific method and the subsequent establishment of accepted community standards of care may suggest uniformity, in reality there is much disagreement in clinical practice. So it is misleading at best to presume, as the bucket metaphor encourages us to do, a stringent *a priori* symmetry between particular treatments and particular medical conditions.

Second, the metaphor assumes that there is agreement about what constitutes a leak in the bucket, or an inherent defect in the treatment. While clinical trials indicate the likely effectiveness and appropriateness of particular treatments for particular medical conditions, the notions of effectiveness and appropriateness are themselves the subject of much disagreement. Obviously, depending on the criteria selected to determine effectiveness and appropriateness, different treatments will be judged differently in different clinical trials.

At issue is not some measurable, inherent quality of a given treatment, but the relationship between the treatment and its proposed application. The proposed application, not the treatment alone, will define the nature of potential leaks. The relationship between the bucket and the condition in need of treatment must be addressed for discussion of the leak to have any relevance.[5]

Third, the metaphor presumes that all leaks are ruinous and ultimately irreparable. In other words, appeals to the metaphor imply that once a leak or inherent defect is identified, the bucket or treatment should be abandoned, as it could never be put to any reasonable use. Furthermore, use of the metaphor seems to lead to the belief that no patches exist that might sufficiently correct bucket or treatment leaks, enabling them to achieve limited and perhaps different ends.

For example, the metaphor does not admit the possibility that vessels not permanently and inherently airtight might still be purposeful. Perhaps a traveler (or patient) only expects or desires the vessel (or treatment) to retain some modest degree of water for a limited amount of time. The vessel (or treatment), especially if patched sufficiently, might capably serve that purpose. Or, maybe the traveler (or patient) simply wishes to walk or continue to exist with the vessel's (or treatment's) assistance, despite its inability to permanently alter the traveler's path (or the patient's ultimate clinical course). In that case, the fact that the bucket has a leak might be less relevant.

Obviously, all presumptions underlying the bucket metaphor are subject to criticism. And they are directly challenged in the contemporary futility debate. In the context of disagreement about these fundamental presumptions, I question the practice of unilaterally refusing to provide treatment on the grounds of futility.

Goals, Not Leaks, Should Define the Meaning of Futility

In light of the disagreement that persists over the accuracy and legitimacy of the bucket metaphor and its underlying presumptions, the etymological roots of futility cannot serve to adjudicate among the variety of meanings and definitions ascribed to the concept of futility or to the normative positions represented in the literature.

A more helpful starting place is Stuart Youngner's early suggestion that we begin by understanding that futility is an instrumental concept. Youngner explains that to understand the meaning of futility in a specific clinical situation, "we must first examine the potential goals of the medical intervention in question."[6] The focus is less on the inherent qualities of, or defects in, the intervention, and more on the uses to which the intervention will be put.

When futility is understood to be linked inextricably to goals, it becomes clear that treatments are never inherently futile, futile *per se*, or futile with respect to everything. Rather, treatments can only be judged futile in relation to the particular goals which they are intended to achieve and for which they can be used as instruments.

Unfortunately, explicit mention and defense of the goals according to which particular treatments are judged futile seldom occurs. Instead, it is far more common for clinicians to make incomplete statements like, "Transfusing this patient would be futile," "Maintaining this patient on a ventilator would be futile," "Dialyzing this patient would be futile," or "Resuscitating these kinds of patients would be futile."

But these statements are meaningless. In each instance, the sentence must be completed to be meaningful. So, "Transfusing this patient is futile" can become meaningful and informative when we add, ". . . with respect to the goal of curing the underlying disease process."

An apt grammatical analogue for the common use of the word futility is, "This ball is not hard enough."[7] While this phrase is technically a complete sentence, it is not meaningful. What's missing is typically missing from futility statements as well: explicit acknowledgment of the presumed referent. The reader is left asking, "Isn't hard enough for what?" or, in the case of futility statements, "Futile with respect to what and to whose goal(s)?"

It would thus be valuable in the clinical setting to insist that the word futility always be used in full sentences, in order to establish a specific context of meaning. Rather than accepting the typical incomplete form in which futility judgments are made, clinicians can clarify the intended meaning and use of the word by asking, "futile with respect to what goal(s) and whose goal(s) is that?"

Because there is no single accepted completion to the statements about futility and no single goal applicable to all medical interventions and to all patients at all times, appeals to futility in the clinical setting often obscure rather than illuminate the essential values and interests at stake in clinical decisions. Clarifying which and whose goals are at issue is one way of identifying and exposing the sources of conflict that characterize debates about futility.

Another useful intervention derives from the recognition that the descriptive and normative meanings of futility are frequently conflated. Much like use of the word "bad," the word "futile" is typically used in a sentence both to describe a quality of a particular treatment and to argue normatively against its use. It is important to insist that if the word "futile" is used, the presuppositions made on the descriptive and normative level must be exposed, and sources of potential conflict at these levels must be acknowledged. I explore the relationship between these descriptive and normative aspects of futility in the chapters that follow.

For now I will only note that even if each of these recommended interventions is made, much more information and argumentation is needed to determine normatively whether treatment described as futile should be provided or foregone.

The Search for a Definition: Possible Treatment Goals

The search for a definition of futility leads to an examination of the goals with respect to which treatments might be deemed futile. A variety of goals have been offered in the contemporary futility literature. To explain the nature of the current debate, I will review the meanings and definitions ascribed to the concept of futility in the most commonly cited articles on the topic. I will identify the explicit goals with respect to which interventions have been considered futile, and then organize the explicitly and implicitly proposed goals into more manageable categories.

Treatments have variously been described as futile if they cannot achieve the goals of: postponing death;[8] prolonging or extending life;[9] improving, maintaining, or restoring quality of life;[10] benefiting the patient;[11] benefiting the patient as a whole;[12] improving prognosis;[13] improving the patient's comfort, well being, or general state of health;[14] reversing or ameliorating an underlying condition;[15] achieving immediate objectives;[16] achieving intended physiologic effects;[17] restoring consciousness;[18] ending dependence on intensive medical care;[19] preventing or curing disease;[20] alleviating suffering; relieving symptoms;[21] restoring function; discharging the patient to home;[22] achieving short or long term survival;[23] achieving the patient's goals;[24] or achieving any of these goals.[25]

This list of potential goals with respect to which treatments could be deemed futile demonstrates the vast disagreement that exists regarding appropriate treatment goals as well as the great potential for conflicts that exists among the goals selected. While a treatment might successfully be employed to achieve a discrete physiologic effect such as restoring electrolyte balance, its use might simultaneously fail to achieve other goals such as preventing death, benefiting the patient as a whole, or maintaining quality of life.

Despite implicit conflicts among the many possible goals of medical interventions, there has yet to be a critical evaluation of their origins, relationships to one another, or acceptable applications. When the goals are referenced in the literature, they are presented as if they are self-evident *a priori* truths, not strategic choices open to challenge from alternative perspectives. Consequently, few if any arguments are presented in favor of selected goals over competing alternative goals.

Even if the necessary argumentation were offered, consensus regarding the selection of goals with respect to which treatments should always be judged futile would not be forthcoming. There is disagreement regarding the selection of goals precisely because the act of selection itself represents a choice among values about which individuals disagree. For that reason, the search for a uniform formula according to which treatments could be considered futile, or for a single definition of futility itself, is doomed to failure.

Given the plurality of values represented in futility conflicts, at issue is not just the selection of goals, but also the establishment of authority for choosing them. And that is an issue that cannot be addressed by merely stipulating the selection of certain goals over others.

Despite the problems inherent in securing a uniform, universally applicable definition of futility, certain core goals have gained prominence in the futility discussion. They have been most often discussed under three general categories: the traditional goals of medicine, the relevance of quality of life, and the standards for cardiopulmonary resuscitation. I will examine each of these in turn.

Traditional Goals of Medicine

The futility literature is full of references to the traditional goals of medicine, which are variously defined as: maximizing patient benefit while minimizing burden or risk of harm (a contemporary interpretation of the Hippocratic maxim); preserving life; preventing or curing disease; preventing or alleviating suffering; and restoring function, health, or general well-being. Typically, treatments that are seen as consistent with the advancement of these traditional goals of medicine are defined as effective and appropriate; those deemed inconsistent with or outside the bounds of the traditional goals are construed as futile.

Curiously, there is little critical analysis of the traditional goals of medicine themselves, of their justification, or of their superiority to alternative goals. In addition, there is little attention given to the fact that stipulating narrow *a priori* goals for medicine in general, or for specific treatment modalities in particular, may fail to take into account the more nuanced and idiosyncratic goals of patients, or, for that matter, of the general lay population.

For example, stipulating the alleviation of pain and suffering as the goal of medicine, or of particular treatment modalities, may conflict with the goals of a patient for whom suffering has redemptive qualities. Stipulating the preservation of life as the goal of medicine, or of particular treatment modalities, may conflict with a patient for whom the goal is alleviation of suffering. Likewise, the medical profession's understanding of the meaning and goal of medicine may fail to take sufficiently into account the perspective of those whom they more broadly serve: the lay population and society in general.

Schneiderman and Jecker's selection of appropriate objectives for physicians to pursue in accordance with their stipulated definition of the goal of medicine offers an interesting case in point. Schneiderman and Jecker describe their approach to futility as fundamentally patient-centered because they focus not simply on achieving effects but on producing genuine benefit for the patient. As such they define as futile treatments that would be highly unlikely to restore consciousness or end dependence on intensive medical care. In their view, such treatments are futile because they have no reasonable chance of benefitting the patient; providing such treatment would thus be inconsistent with the goals of medicine.[26]

While it may be helpful to distinguish treatment that will produce an effect from treatment that is medically beneficial, the problems of deciding whose perception and definition of "effect" and "benefit" will count, and whose choice of goal is authoritative remain unresolved. Schneiderman and Jecker like to describe their overall approach and selection of goals as patient-centered, but on these key points their model is clearly and unapologetically physician driven. There are a number of problems with this approach.

To begin, stipulating as the sole goal of medicine the achievement of medical benefit is ultimately a tautology. In other words, basing the argument on a stipulation of the goals of medicine begs the most important questions: What is the ultimate source of and justification for the goals of medicine? From what process are the goals of medicine derived and with what participation from which stakeholders? To what degree does the lay population share the medical profession's vision of its appropriate goals, and therefore to what degree should the profession's vision have standing? I take these questions up more fully in Chapter 5. Here it will be sufficient to note the difficulty inherent in any process of selecting the goal of medicine in general or of specific treatment modalities in particular.

Tomlinson and Czlomka begin to pursue this line of inquiry in their critique of Schneiderman and Jecker's selection of the goal of restoration of consciousness and their subsequent judgment that it would be futile to treat patients in a persistent vegetative state.

> Such judgments make assumptions about the proper goals of medicine that have not been validated through broad and open public dialogue. . . . Extending a patient's life, even one of such attenuated quality, is most certainly among the traditional goals of medicine. Without the backdrop of such a tradition, there would have been no need to make any ethical or legal arguments on behalf of terminally ill patients' rights to limit life-

prolonging treatments. A policy that defines futile by reference to permanent unconsciousness, then, departs from this tradition and attempts to change it by fiat. It is a departure, however, that at this stage in our history does not have the clear warrant of broad social agreement.[27]

In fact, there is little empirical evidence to support Schneiderman and Jecker's claim that their selection of the goal of restoration of consciousness is supported widely,[28] or that their definition of "benefit" is shared generally.

If society is to have a meaningful role in sanctioning professional standards of practice, it would seem that these questions need considered public reflection and debate. Unfortunately, the role Schneiderman and Jecker describe for society seems to be more reactive than directive. They define medically futile treatments as treatments that fail to advance the goals of medicine in that they offer no benefit to the patient above a minimal quantitative or qualitative threshhold. Within these parameters, they call on the medical profession to work first to reach internal consensus as to which treatments fail to achieve the goals of medicine, and only thereafter to seek society's concurrence.[29]

Ironically, while Schneiderman and Jecker acknowledge a need for public support and consensus, they seem to introduce it only after the fact, when all of the most important normative choices have already been made. They concede that their use of the term "goals of medicine" is normative, and that the impetus for their book *Wrong Medicine* is "a desire to restore a vision of medicine's proper ends and reform medical practice."[30] But it seems that public participation is invited only within the confines of this already constructed and carefully predefined frame of reference. What is missing, of course, is a meaningful opportunity to question the medical profession's normative interpretation of the appropriate goals and vision of medicine itself.

Quality of Life

A related body of literature that illustrates the significance of selecting some goals and not others centers on the explicit discussion of quality of life. Judgments about quality of life take a variety of forms. Concern can be centered on maintaining a patient's existing quality of life, restoring previous quality of life, or improving quality of life. Depending on which variation of the goal is selected, proposed treatments may or may not be judged futile.

Apart from the issue of selecting which variation of the goal of quality of life to accomplish, there is the equally vexing problem of defining quality of life itself. While the literature on futility, and on bioethics in general, is replete with references to quality of life, the concept itself remains elusive and ill-defined.

Though there has been a movement to develop measurements for and indicators of quality of life,[31] none of us can legitimately claim to know truly and authoritatively what another's quality of life is. While we may be in a position to make observations about an individual's external presentation, unless we are living in her body and in her interior world of experience, we cannot claim to know how she perceives or values the quality of her existence.[32] For this reason, it is argued, only patients themselves are in a position to provide reliable and meaningful information about their own quality of life. And in fact, recent studies have documented the frank inability of health care providers and family members to know accurately how patients actually assess their own quality of life.[33] Nonetheless, despite the problems inherent in quality of life judgments, the impulse to offer only those treatments that will maintain, restore, or improve quality of life resonates throughout the contemporary futility discussion.

This has been demonstrated with respect to the goal of restoring consciousness. Interestingly, neurological status is one aspect of quality of life that has become central to the futility discussion. As I have indicated, arguments are presented frequently, on the grounds of futility, against sustaining the lives of patients in a persistent vegetative state. The focus on consciousness and the capacity for relationality as primary goals is not new. The court opinion in the Karen Ann Quinlan case underscored the importance of consciousness by questioning whether Ms. Quinlan would ever return to a "cognitive sapient state."[34] Early comments on the treatment of handicapped infants frequently stipulated the importance of the potential for relationality with others and with the surrounding environment.[35]

Most recently, discussion has focused on the specific meaning and worth of life in a persistent vegetative state. Like Schneiderman and Jecker, Jecker and Robert A. Pearlman assert the popularity of one particular perspective on the matter.

[M]ost people would agree that qualities such as consciousness, self-consciousness, and the ability to communicate must be part of a minimally meaningful existence.[36]

Again, the question is whether the assessments of health care professionals accurately reflect the perspective of the society at large. Clearly stories like Helga Wanglie's[37] offer examples of a patient's disagreement with the formulation and imposition of the goal of consciousness. Obviously, stipulating the restoration of consciousness as the goal of medicine, or of particular treatment modalities, may conflict with a patient for whom the goal is preservation of life irrespective of its quality. Again, the notion that consciousness is a part of a minimally meaningful existence is not an *a priori* universalizable truth.

Weighing the importance of consciousness is but one aspect of judging whether a particular treatment will be successful in achieving the goal of maintaining, restoring, or improving quality of life. And, of course, judging whether a particular treatment will be successful in achieving the goal of maintaining, restoring, or improving quality of life is but one aspect of determining whether or not the proposed treatment is futile.

Standards for Cardiopulmonary Resuscitation (CPR)

A final source of goals that have been influential in advancing the futility debate can be found in the evolution of standards for cardiopulmonary resuscitation (CPR). Discussion about the medical indications for CPR has introduced the idea that the goal against which this intervention's success or failure should be measured is discharge to home. In other words, if an attempted resuscitation eventually results in the patient's being discharged to home, the attempt will be judged in retrospect to have been a success. If the attempted resuscitation does not eventually result in the patient being discharged to home, the attempt will be judged in retrospect to have been a failure.

Several articles have used this goal as the standard by which success and failure are measured, in order to demonstrate that resuscitation is medically futile and therefore contraindicated for certain kinds of patients, specifically: the elderly;[38] patients with renal failure,[39] pneumonia,[40] cancer,[41] or sepsis;[42] babies with very low birth weights;[43] and patients who arrest outside of the hospital.[44]

Though discharge to home could be challenged as an essentially arbitrary and narrow goal, it enjoys widespread acceptance in the literature. Clearly the leading articles on CPR would have a different flavor, and would reach different conclusions, if the goal of resuscitation were restoration of heartbeat, or continued short-term in-hospital survival, or even improved cardiovascular health.

Some have extrapolated to other medical interventions the reasoning behind the selection of discharge to home as the goal of CPR. For example, Schneiderman, Jecker, and Jonsen, and Schneiderman and Jecker suggest that if a patient will be forever dependent on intensive medical treatment, such treatment should be defined as futile.[45] But by rejecting goals that may be inconsistent with their vision of independent functioning, the authors exclude goals, such as continued existence, that may be in accord with the patient's own goals and value system.

The CPR literature, and the discussion it has spawned, are notable examples of how the selection of goals influences judgments about an intervention's effectiveness and appropriateness. They also demonstrate how the selection of goals is itself a value choice. Both of these points resurface as significant features of the contemporary futility discussion.

Goals and the Classic Formulations of Futility Appeals

Once the possible goals with respect to which treatments could be judged futile are grouped into these categories, at least one more observation can be made about them. The goals against which a treatment will be judged futile, as well as the meaning and weight ascribed to the goals themselves, depend upon the formulation of futility used. The term "futility" means that the goal for which the treatment is proposed is either unachievable or insufficiently worthwhile. In the first instance, the treatment is described conventionally as ineffective, or what I have called physiologically or factually futile. In the second instance, the treatment is described customarily as inappropriate, or what I have called evaluatively futile.

According to the approach popularized in the literature, the judgment that a treatment will be ineffective in achieving a designated goal is presumed to be overwhelmingly factual and devoid of significant evaluative content. Judgment that a treatment is physiologically futile implies only that it is not possible physiologically to successfully pursue the goal with respect to which the treatment is futile. Such a judgment does not imply that the goal is not worth pursuing. Conversely, judgment that a treatment is evaluatively futile is recognized commonly to reflect and to derive from the values of the individual making the judgment. Such a judgment does not describe some objective fact about the relationship between the treatment and the goal, much less about the possibility of the treatment's successful use as an instrument of a goal. An evaluative judgment of futility indicates only that the goal itself would not be worth pursuing, not that the treatment would be an ineffective instrument in achieving the goal. The two classic formulations of futility offer unique perspectives from which treatments and goals can be evaluated. From a factual perspective, we can investigate whether the treatment in question is a possible means of achieving the designated goal. From an evaluative perspective, we can judge the worthiness of a designated goal and hence the worthiness of employing the treatment as a means of achieving it.

The debate about resuscitation standards nicely illustrates this point. We can evaluate whether or not an attempted resuscitation would be futile through two discrete lenses. If we are concerned primarily with effectiveness (that is, with whether resuscitation will work physiologically), we can ask whether attempted resuscitation is likely to achieve the goals of restoration of heartbeat or short-term survival. If we are concerned primarily with appropriateness (that is, with whether attempted resuscitation will be worth it), we can ask whether the goals of discharge to home or enhanced quality of life are worth pursuing.

Regardless of the perspective chosen, for a judgment of futility to have meaning in the contemporary discussion, there must be a relationship between the treatment designated as ineffective or inappropriate and the goals that the treatment will allegedly fail to achieve. Once the significance of the selection of goals is established, a number of questions are raised. Who should define and select the goals, and according to what criteria? How should conflicts of definition and criteria be resolved? These questions are at the heart of the futility debate and link the two epistemological questions raised by the problem of futility.

Having explored the etymological roots of futility, as well as the various meanings ascribed to futility and their relationship to the two classic formulations of futility, we can now turn to the equally difficult epistemological problem of establishing acceptable criteria for recognizing ineffective or inappropriate treatments. Even if goals are agreed upon, and a definition of futility is established, criteria will be needed to judge whether particular treatments qualify as futile.

To address the problem of selecting acceptable criteria for recognizing, knowing, or judging treatments to be ineffective from a factual perspective, or inappropriate from an evaluative perspective, I will consider procedural and substantive answers that have been offered in the contemporary discussion. I will give special attention to how the procedural and substantive answers in the standard analysis vary depending upon which classic formulation of futility is at stake.

Criteria for Knowing When Treatments Are Futile

Procedural Approaches

One way of approaching the epistemological problem of setting criteria for recognizing treatments to be factually or evaluatively futile is to focus not on substantive criteria, but on the procedural question of who should be empowered to make such judgments. Authority to recognize a treatment to be ineffective or inappropriate could be assigned exclusively to patients, family members, other appointed surrogates, physicians, nurses, other members of the health care team, hospital administrators, insurers, society, or some combination thereof.

Patients, physicians, society, or some combination thereof figure most prominently in the futility literature's preliminary responses to the limited question of who should be empowered to judge whether particular treatments qualify as physiologically or evaluatively futile.

According to the standard analysis of the procedural question, the privilege and power to make evaluative judgments of futility is generally accorded to patients, while the privilege and power to make factual judgments of futility is generally reserved for physicians. The role of the larger society in setting parameters for such judgments is increasingly the subject of public debate.

At issue in providing a defensible answer to the procedural question is the difficult matter of expertise. If, as the standard analysis suggests, evaluative futility judgments are based on values and factual futility judgments are based on facts, are there such skills as evaluative expertise or factual expertise? Might certain parties to a conflict be more expert in facts and other parties more expert in values? And what should follow procedurally once such expertise is identified? Before exploring these questions, I must clarify my use of the less familiar language of "evaluative expertise."

When I ask who is more expert in the values that inform medical decision making, I am asking not who is more expert in the values that ought to always and universally guide decision making, but rather who is more expert in the particular personal values that guide patients' approach to illness and medical decision making. I am not, therefore, asking whether patients have any more expertise in general matters of values than physicians, or even whether such expertise is actually possible. Further, I am not arguing that expertise is a necessary condition of decision making authority.

Patient Expertise

Most of the bioethics literature in general, and the futility literature in particular, presumes that in conflicts between patients and physicians, patients are more expert in evaluative matters that have direct consequences for their lives and bodies, and physicians are more expert in factual scientific matters. Following that general bias, many contributors[46] to the futility literature have suggested that patients are in the best position to select therapeutic goals and to judge whether they are worth achieving. Accordingly, they are in the best position to evaluate, interpret, and weigh available medical information and to make evaluative judgments about whether a particular treatment modality is appropriate and worth trying. This is generally accepted as true because only patients know how much risk they are willing to endure and how much they value particular benefits.[47] As Charles Fried puts it, each individual patient has a unique "risk budget." Patients calculate

> In rough ways, out of their experience, emotions, and energy, the extent of security and danger they will accept in their lives.[48]

And patients alone live with the outcomes of medical interventions. From this perspective, patients are thus always in the best position to recognize when treatments are evaluatively futile for them (that is, not worth trying). At the very least, they should be significantly involved in making such determinations. Seldom are patients considered sufficiently expert to make judgments about the probability of a treatment's success in achieving their desired goal.

Physician Expertise

The standard analysis presumes that when it comes to gathering and interpreting the empirical data and evaluating its relevance for a given patient, physicians are more expert than patients. For that reason, many authors[49] have argued that physicians are in the best position to recognize authoritatively when therapeutic goals cannot be achieved and when treatments are ineffective. Only physicians, it is argued, have the knowledge and expertise to recognize when they are confronted with physiologically futile treatments. It is therefore ultimately the physician's responsibility to assess the clinical facts and to recognize when treatment modalities will be ineffective in achieving designated goals.

For the most part, authors sympathetic to this position are careful to limit the physician's authority to making judgments of factual futility. Elaborating on the distinction between quantitative and qualitative futility initially made by Schneiderman, Jecker, and Jonsen,[50] Jecker and Pearlman argue that

> Authority to render a judgment about quantitative futility rests squarely with physicians. . . . [I]t is physicians who are responsible for determining whether their patients meet the conditions.[51]

Others are less clear about limits, and allow for the possibility that physicians may make judgments of evaluative futility as well as factual futility.

> The physician must be careful not to offer ICU care once there is no reasonable chance it will improve outcome. . . . The difficulty arises when the patient's prognosis is unclear. It is ethically appropriate for the physician as the patient's advocate to interpret the clinical information and advise the patient and family whether intensive care will be beneficial. . . . [T]his is ultimately the physician's responsibility.[52]

Assigning to physicians the tasks of deciding both whether a treatment will improve the chances for a desired outcome and whether it will be beneficial presents a host of normative problems that I take up in the chapters to follow.

The Societal Context

Of course, patients and physicians do not make evaluative or factual judgments of futility in a vacuum. Perhaps there is a larger role for society to play in setting the parameters within which judgments of futility can be made. A possible modification to the position that patients be given latitude to decide that a goal or treatment is not worth pursuing is to place greater emphasis on the needs of the community and on consensus about collective priorities. If there is broad community consensus that certain outcomes and certain existences (for example, life in a persistent vegetative state) are below a minimally acceptable threshold, perhaps a greater burden of proof and a greater financial responsibility could be imposed upon patients who insist on making evaluative judgments contrary to shared communal values and priorities.[53] If we extend this thought to its natural conclusion, we can perhaps conclude that patients should only have latitude to make evaluative judgments of futility in instances when community consensus does not exist. Examples of such situations that have been suggested are ventilator dependency for conscious patients or treatment for patients with end-stage acute myelogenous leukemia.[54]

A possible modification to the position that physicians be given latitude to decide that a goal is not achievable or a treatment is ineffective might be to open to public debate the criteria by which effectiveness is measured and by which the acceptable probabilities of error are determined.[55] I take up this possibility more directly in Chapter 5.

Many who think and write about the problem of futility hope that the growing body of literature itself may lead society to develop consensual criteria by which to judge potentially futile treatments. In Chapter 5, I also discuss further how public discourse and resultant social consensus might resolve some of the epistemological and normative problems at the heart of many of the most difficult futility conflicts.

Substantive Approaches

No matter *who* is assigned the task of recognizing whether or not particular treatments qualify as evaluatively or factually futile, the challenge remains of establishing *how* such judgments can be made.

As part of my conceptual analysis of the meanings and uses of appeals to futility, I have deliberately distinguished procedural and substantive approaches to the epistemological problem of establishing criteria for recognizing futile treatments. While we may be tempted to presume a traditional and direct correspondence between who makes the determination and how the determination is made, such a simplistic characterization would fail to take into account the complexity of the task and the sophistication of those elected to perform it. Patients, physicians, and society may each appeal to any of the available substantive approaches in deciding whether particular treatments qualify as futile.

There are at least two distinct ways to respond substantively to the epistemological problem of establishing criteria for recognizing treatments as futile. Judgments may draw on informational sources, such as anecdotes, clinical judgment, or statistical evidence, or they may derive from theoretical frameworks, such as principle-driven or casuistical approaches. Though specific informational sources and specific theoretical approaches may be associated in practice, they are not necessarily related. For that reason, I will consider briefly each of these substantive criteria. I will also note whether the standard analysis considers each possible kind of substantive criteria more or less relevant for making judgments of evaluative and factual futility.

Informational Sources

ANECDOTAL INFORMATION Physicians, patients, and the broader society may all rely on anecdotal information in assessing whether particular treatments qualify as futile or not in both the evaluative and factual sense. Anecdotal information often influences whether treatments are judged as appropriate from an evaluative perspective, and effective from a physiological or factual perspective.

Memory of an outlier case, an unexpected recovery, or a disastrous outcome can influence which features of a new clinical situation are noticed and which are passed over, which studies are considered relevant, which risks are deemed worth taking, and therefore which particular treatment options are judged futile. For physicians and patients alike, past experiences certainly shape hopes, fears, desires, and expectations. This phenomenon is borne out daily in clinical practice and decision making.[56]

One telling case in point is a *New York Times* article[57] describing an influential report in the *New England Journal of Medicine*. The report, by William A. Gray and his colleagues at Brown University, regarded the futility of bringing patients to the hospital after an unsuccessful attempt at resuscitation in the field.[58] The retrospective study documents that only 16 of 185 patients who arrived in the emergency room after an initially unsuccessful resuscitation attempt in the field were revived ultimately and admitted to the hospital. None survived to be discharged to home; all but one were comatose throughout their hospitalizations. The authors conclude that emergency room resuscitative efforts with patients for whom prehospital resuscitation has failed is neither an effective nor a worthwhile expenditure of communal resources.

The article reports several physicians' comments on the study. One cardiologist admits that, though the study is impressive, he "would hate to give up on patients because, occasionally, someone survives." A colleague concurs because he "knew of one man who was revived in the hospital after an emergency team had failed to resuscitate him and who lived to leave the hospital." In this case, even though the evidence suggested that resuscitation of such patients is ineffective, anecdotal information seemed to contradict this evidence, and shaped the physicians' evaluative judgments of whether the intervention would be worth trying.[59] Patients are similarly swayed by the power of anecdotal information, especially when treatment options represent a choice between life or death.

The tendency to weight anecdotal information heavily, even in the face of substantiated epidemiological data, significantly influences whether particular treatments are judged to be futile. Separate and apart from statistical evidence, anecdotal information can influence any participant in the decision making process to view particular treatment options as futile in either of the two classic senses of the word. Anecdotal information can persuade patients, family members, other surrogates, physicians, or society to judge treatments to be either ineffective from a factual perspective or inappropriate from an evaluative perspective.

CLINICAL JUDGMENT Alternatively, anyone positioned to make a futility judgment may be influenced by the repository of accumulated clinical experience that leads to what we call clinical judgment. Though clinical judgment is primarily associated with clinicians, lay members of a health care community may have their own sense of how to recognize effective or appropriate treatments, based on their accumulated clinical experiences. At issue is not so much who has clinical judgment but what the meaning, source, and weight of the judgment should be.

The appeal to sustained firsthand clinical experience as the worthiest basis of decision making has a long history.[60] Applied to the contemporary futility debate, clinical judgment might serve as a substantive criterion for determining whether the goal of a particular treatment is achievable and sufficiently worthwhile. That clinical judgment might serve as the basis for either kind of futility judgment suggests that clinical judgment has both a factual and an evaluative component. This is one of the many aspects of clinical judgment that has received insufficient attention in the current discussion.

The argument typically made in favor of clinical judgment as a means of determining futility is that clinicians are in a privileged epistemic position. They have immediate access to the complicated body of information and experience that proves most instructive when difficult judgments and decisions must be made. Clinicians' developed intuition and vast experience allows them to judge most meaningfully the likelihood of a particular treatment succeeding or failing for a patient with a particular history as well as the likelihood of the patient benefitting from the intervention.

It is not just that they went to medical school and have a body of technical information at their disposal. The finest physicians develop a gestalt sense of how to best treat their patients. This is one part of the art of medicine. Knowing which patients will make it and can be helped, and which will die despite everyone's best efforts, comes from years of accumulated clinical experience.

The weight given to clinical judgment is strongly supported in the literature. One example of this is the documentation of physicians' ability to predict accurately which of their patients will die during hospitalization.[61] Of course, predictions are never completely accurate. But the accuracy of predictions grounded in clinical judgment cannot be denied. According to the accepted approach, the body of accumulated clinical experience called clinical judgment is the best source of information about what diagnostic, prognostic, and therapeutic interventions are not only possible, but also legitimate for particular patients.

Many physicians are convinced that their clinical judgment entitles them to make not only judgments of ineffectiveness from a factual perspective, but also judgments of inappropriateness from an evaluative perspective. This is one of the questions I take up in the chapters that follow.

Though many contributors to the futility literature portray clinical judgment as the most appropriate and reliable basis for judgments of futility, the notion of clinical judgment itself presents problems. While it is considered a reliable disinterested source for objective value-free standards of medical indications and contraindications, clinical judgment varies significantly across the clinician population.

Sociological studies have identified factors that may affect clinical judgment and decision making. These include patient characteristics, clinician characteristics, clinician interaction with the medical profession and the larger health care system, and the clinician-patient relationship.[62] An important study confirmed the power and potential bias of clinical judgment, over and above documented prognostic data, by finding that patients with AIDS or lung cancer were more likely to receive DNR orders than patients with cirrhosis or severe congestive heart failure.[63] The authors of the study theorized that, though the patients had similar prognoses, physicians perceived the patients differently and made different clinical judgments about the appropriateness of a DNR order depending on the underlying disease. Obviously the question is whether this was a reasonable exercise of differing clinical judgment, or whether non-medical factors resulted in an unwarranted inequity in the care of patients.

In short, no one doubts that health care professionals make clinical judgments based on accumulated knowledge and experience that far exceeds that of the typical member of the lay public. At issue is the extent to which such knowledge and experience should be determinative, and whether it should be accorded different weight when it is used to ground judgments of physiologic futility or evaluative futility.

STATISTICAL EVIDENCE Statistical evidence about probable outcomes is a third substantive measure of whether particular treatments qualify as futile. According to the standard analysis, statistical evidence can best be used to prove that a particular treatment is effective or ineffective for achieving a specified goal. By tracking utility, benefit, effectiveness, harm, and risk, statistical evidence offers the hope of quantifying intuitive experience-based clinical judgments of futility and providing clear guidance on which course of action would be most likely to achieve the desired results.

Espousing a position that combines clinical judgment and statistical evidence, Schneiderman, Jecker, and Jonsen propose that

> [W]hen physicians conclude (either through personal experience, experiences shared with colleagues, or consideration of reported empiric data) that in the last 100 cases, a medical treatment has been useless, they should regard that treatment as futile.[64]

According to an approach that relies on statistical evidence, the best way to determine whether a particular treatment qualifies as futile is to conduct and rely upon controlled empirical studies, including randomized, prospective, multicenter clinical trials. The literature already provides a number of studies that assess not only the effectiveness but also the appropriateness of specific medical interventions for particular patient populations based on outcome studies. The articles referenced earlier that report survival for different categories of patients after intensive care or attempted CPR are excellent examples of this growing body of influential studies.

Another related body of literature comes from the outcomes movement itself and from the move to quantify prognostic indicators. Dubbed by Arnold S. Relman "the third revolution in medical care,"[65] the outcomes movement has refocussed clinical judgment and decision making from in-dividual clinicians' judgments of individual patients to statistical evidence.

Proponents of the outcomes movement identify as its three most impor-tant goals: increasing knowledge of the effectiveness of different interven-tions, enhancing decision making by clinicians and patients, and develop-ing standards to guide clinicians and assist third-party payers in selecting cost-effective treatments.[66] Manifestations of the outcomes movement can be found in the Joint Commission on the Accreditation of Healthcare Or-ganization's (JCAHO) adoption of quality assessment based on severity-adjusted outcomes, in the Health Care Financing Administration's (HCFA) program aimed at measuring effectiveness and generating guidelines for practice based on outcomes,[67] and in the establishment of the federal Agency for Health Care Policy and Research (especially its Medical Treat-ment and Effectiveness Program, which funds studies of patient outcomes and treatment alternatives, as well as optimal treatment for specific condi-tions).[68]

Probably more than anyone else, William A. Knaus and his colleagues have contributed to the development and increasing use of prognostic indi-cators and outcomes studies in clinical judgment and decision making. By introducing a severity-of-disease classification system called APACHE (Acute Physiology, Age, and Chronic Health Evaluation) in the early 1980s, they hoped to offer an objective tool for clinicians to use in estimating prog-nosis and in selecting reasonable therapeutic options.

Already in its third version, the APACHE system uses a severity-of-disease model to offer reference data to ICU clinicians who treat patients with acute organ-system failure. The computer-based APACHE III system correlates individual patient information with a database of prognostic in-formation collected from 17,440 adults admitted to medical or surgical ICUs around the country. The APACHE system is designed to measure and score an individual patient's likelihood of death or survival upon admission to an ICU and twice during each day. At each step in clinical decision making, systems like APACHE enable "an individual clinician [to] have the collec-tive experience of having treated thousands of similar patients."[69]

The data from outcome studies and systems like APACHE[70] are used fre-quently to establish that certain treatments are futile for patients with cer-tain conditions. Arguing in favor of an objective statistical approach to establishing substantive criteria for the evaluation of treatment options, Knaus and his colleagues assert that

Anchoring [prognostic] estimates with valid and reliable morbidity and
mortality estimates [is] especially useful in mitigating the individual physician's subjective bias or inexperience.... Use of [objective probability
estimates] would increase the precision of communication by reducing re-
liance on emotional, poorly calibrated, and routinely misunderstood qualitative descriptors such as "hopeless," "unsalvageable," and "terminal."[71]

Countering the popular trend of relying heavily on APACHE scores in
planning treatment, Knaus and his colleagues are careful to note that the
APACHE system can only offer information about one piece of the futility
equation.

Decision-making about an individual patient should, to the greatest extent
possible, adopt the patient's view of the relative desirability of various outcome states. Defining futility regarding future therapy requires both objective probability estimates and an evaluative judgment in setting the threshold.... Objective estimates [must not] be misunderstood as decision rules.
... Objective probability estimates will not resolve most ethical controversies.[72]

Anticipating similar potential misuses of epidemiological and statistical methods for determining whether particular treatments should be offered to particular patients, Jonsen reminds us that though clinicians may
be tempted to use statistics "to steer clear of dangerous or inefficacious
treatment, ... any particular patient is a statistic of one."[73] Any single patient's actual prognosis can never be reflected conclusively by statistical
estimations.

Similarly, while Schneiderman, Jecker, and Jonsen propose that we define
as futile any treatment that has not achieved its appointed goal in the previous 100 cases, a simple understanding of statistics will lead necessarily to
the recognition that it is impossible to conclude based on evidence from 100
previous cases what will happen exactly in the 101st case. Rather than ex-
pecting retrospective statistical evidence to lead to accurate prospective predictions, we should recognize that it can only lead to probability statements
subject to an array of influences.[74]

Despite these cautions, statistically-based systems for determining
whether particular treatments qualify as physiologically or evaluatively futile remain enormously appealing to practicing clinicians. I return to the
problems with the popular approach to statistics in the chapters that follow.

In summary, anecdotal information, clinical judgment, and statistical evidence are three sources of information that may be used to respond substantively to the epistemological problem of establishing criteria for recognizing treatments as physiologically or evaluatively futile. Another substantive approach might be adopted as well.

Theoretical Frameworks

Though considerably less has been written about this second source of substantive criteria, a more theoretical approach might be adopted to identify potentially futile treatments. Instead of reviewing all of the possible theoretical frameworks for recognizing futile treatments, I will restrict my focus to the established methodologies of principle-based and casuistic or case-based approaches. While explaining how each might generate substantive criteria for judging treatments to be futile, I will also note some of the more obvious challenges each of these approaches has to face.

PRINCIPLE-BASED APPROACH Rather than rehearse their philosophical origins and justification, I will merely identify the hallmark principles of bioethics: beneficence, nonmaleficence, respect for autonomy, and justice. Though debate exists regarding their appropriate relationship to each other,[75] and regarding the usefulness of their application, the principles themselves have been enormously influential in framing ethical reflection and discussion. For that reason, contributors to the contemporary futility debate frequently address the problem of futility from a perspective of explicit or implicit allegiance to one or more of the principles of bioethics. And they typically assume that one or more of the principles carry greater moral weight than the others when conflicts around futility arise.

Because the principles of bioethics figure so prominently in the futility literature, it is important to note the influence they have on the determination of whether treatments qualify as physiologically or evaluatively futile. For those who subscribe to the principle-based approach, treatments could be judged futile if they comply with and successfully advance the hallmark principles of bioethics. In such a way the principles themselves could become the substantive criteria for identifying treatments as futile.

So, for example, if beneficence is used as a criterion, only treatments that fail to benefit patients will be deemed futile. If nonmaleficence is used as a criterion, only treatments that fail to minimize or avoid harm to patients will be deemed futile. If autonomy is used as a criterion, only treatments that violate the patient's own self-determination will be deemed futile. If justice is used as a criterion, only treatments that fail to serve the interests of fairness and equity will be deemed futile.

Obviously, this approach to selecting substantive criteria for judging treatments to be futile is not without its problems. While it supplies helpful categories for evaluating treatments, the principle-based approach can be highly simplistic and ultimately unhelpful in resolving conflicts. In most theories the principles provide no means of adjudicating conflicts among themselves.[76] Additionally, a treatment's status as futile under the principle-based approach depends upon the principle or principles selected as primary, upon the interpretations of the principles adopted, upon the measurement used to determine whether the underlying values are advanced, and upon the justification provided for each of these choices. Because there is persistent debate at all of these levels, the principle-based approach, while initially appealing, might ultimately prove unsatisfactory as a source of substantive criteria for judging treatments to be futile.

CASUISTRY-BASED APPROACH Casuistry is another methodology that might be adopted as a substantive measure of whether a particular treatment qualifies as futile.[77] Using a case-based approach to the identification of futile treatments, a casuist would seek to uncover the morally relevant features of the particular case. An attempt would be made to situate the case in a taxonomy of similar cases in which the question of futility might be raised. Rejecting a deductive, principle-based approach to the determination of futility, a casuist would attempt to reason inductively from the details of the specific case to a normative judgment about how it ought to be handled. And the casuistic method would encourage reasoning across cases in the taxonomy.

For example, a casuist might identify treatment of brain dead patients as a paradigmatic case of medically ineffective and inappropriate treatment and treatment of pneumonia patients free of other underlying conditions as a paradigmatic case of medically effective and appropriate treatment. When confronted with a dilemma over whether to treat a patient in a persistent vegetative state, the casuist would begin by considering whether treating such a patient would be more like treating the brain dead patient or more like treating the patient with pneumonia. The focus would be on identifying the morally relevant features of each case that make it like and unlike other cases that have been considered.

Like the principle-based approach, casuistry presents problems. Casuistic methodology does not provide answers to the questions of how to determine the morally relevant features of cases, or how to weigh features that are uncovered. And the casuistic method lacks guiding principles that might provide instruction in cases of seemingly irreconcilable conflict.

As substantive alternatives to the problem of establishing criteria for deeming treatments futile, both the principle-based and casuistic approaches may incorporate any of the informational sources discussed earlier. One way to judge whether using a particular treatment is consistent with either approach would be to gather information from anecdotes, clinical judgment, and statistical evidence. The informational sources and theoretical frameworks could be used together to craft substantive criteria for judging treatments to be futile. A review of the contemporary futility literature reveals that many combinations of these alternatives have been promoted as substantive criteria.

That such a wide variety of approaches to the establishment and use of subtantive criteria are referenced in the literature illustrates the degree to which disagreement persists. Just as there is no consensus regarding appropriate definitions and goals, so too there is no consensus regarding acceptable substantive criteria for the recognition of evaluatively or factually futile treatments. This failure to establish consensually agreed upon answers to the epistemological problems of defining futility and establishing criteria by which it can be recognized raises serious questions about the legitimacy of the normative position that supports physician unilateral refusal to provide requested treatment on the grounds of futility. That physicians are in the best position to make futility judgments and that they employ the best substantive criteria has yet to be established.

Summary

The purpose of this chapter has been to fill a gap in the existing discussion of futility by offering a conceptual analysis of the term itself. I have considered two critical epistemological questions raised by the concept of futility. First, to address the problem of identifying the definition and meaning of futility, I have considered the etymological roots of futility, noting the limitations inherent in such an analysis. Having explained the relevance of goals to any definition of futility, I have explored various goals that have been associated with the concept of futility in the contemporary literature. Second, to address the problem of selecting criteria according to which futile treatments could be recognized or known, I have considered the procedural and substantive answers that have been offered.

This chapter has identified the conceptual questions in need of clarification before the concept of futility can be used in a meaningful, appropriate, or useful way. It has revealed the absence of a consensually agreed upon answer to either of the two epistemological questions. Though the literature on futility is extensive, there is ultimately no agreement on *the* definition and meaning of futility, or on the range of acceptable definitions and meanings. Similarly, though the literature is full of normative proposals for what should follow once a judgment of futility is made, there is no agreement on the criteria by which treatments should be judged futile.

It is not surprising that there is disagreement over the correct or acceptable answers to the fundamental epistemological questions raised by futility. Definition and selection of criteria are inherently value-laden choices. There is disagreement about proper definition and criteria precisely because there is disagreement about the moral weight of the underlying values at stake.

It is in the context of this profound disagreement that the normative arguments about what should follow from futility judgments must be much more carefully evaluated. The next two chapters take up this normative question by considering whether either classic formulation of futility, as currently developed, is sufficient to justify unilateral refusal to provide treatment. Chapter 3 considers futility appeals made on the grounds that treatment would be inappropriate (that is, would not be worth it). Chapter 4 considers futility appeals made on the grounds that treatment would be ineffective (that is, would not work). In each instance I examine how the appeal to futility is formulated and evaluate whether it is sufficient to justify physician unilateral refusal to provide treatment.

A QUESTION OF VALUES
The Problem with Evaluative Futility

WHEN THE CONCEPT of futility is used as a decision making tool in the policy arena or in the clinical setting, there are many sources of potential conflicts. Only against the backdrop of these very real but as yet unresolved conflicts can the normative arguments in favor of physician unilateral decision making on the grounds of futility be evaluated meaningfully.

On one level, conflicts may persist over the definitions and meanings of futility, as well as over the criteria for recognition. On another level, conflicts may persist about who has the requisite expertise, who should be empowered to select the goals with respect to which treatments may be judged futile, and how those empowered with selection should select the criteria for recognizing treatments as futile. On a final level, even if conflicts of definition and criteria are resolved, conflicts may still persist over what should follow normatively from a judgment that a particular treatment is futile for a particular patient.

Conflicts over Evaluative Futility

In the cases that follow, I describe three different scenarios, two in which a patient or family disagree with a physician's judgment of evaluative futility, and one in which a physician avoids a potential conflict over evaluative futility by choosing conversation rather than unilateral decision making. Each case illustrates possible implications of granting physicians authority to unilaterally refuse to offer, provide, or continue treatment on the grounds of evaluative futility. In the first case, the physician's judgment of evaluative futility is based only on his personal beliefs and prejudices. In the second case, the physician's judgment of evaluative futility is based on his assessment of professional standards and an emerging societal consensus. In the final case, the physician gives the patient an opportunity to influence his determination of whether the treatment in question is evaluatively futile.

Clinical Examples of Allegedly Evaluative Futility

Case Report #1[1]

A 34-year-old woman with a longstanding history of alcoholism and alcoholic liver disease presented to a community hospital with complaints of having vomited blood. She had had tarry stools for two weeks.

Her medical history was notable for a hospitalization one year prior for delirium tremens, alcoholic hepatitis, hemorrhagic gastritis, hemorrhagic duodenitis, and esophageal varices.

In the emergency room, the patient admitted to typically drinking one and a half quarts of alcohol a day, though for the past few days she had limited her intake to two or three glasses of wine a day. When contacted by the emergency room physician, her physician of record stated that he had previously discharged the patient from his practice due to persistent drinking.

After being evaluated in the emergency room, the patient was admitted to the ICU for transfusion therapy and control of delirium tremens. Despite transfusion therapy, which itself was complicated due to the patient's rare blood type, the patient continued to bleed. A surgical consultation indicated that in view of her coagulopathy and overall poor prognosis, the patient would not survive the needed total gastrectomy. Intensive support was continued. The patient's condition waxed and waned. For a few days she was unresponsive and had rapid breathing. Eventually, her condition stabilized and she was transferred to the Med-Surg unit where her level of alertness improved. She required a paracentesis to remove one liter of fluid. While she had no further exsanguination, she continued to slowly bleed. Her hepatic function continued to deteriorate.

Her treating physician sought guidance from the bioethics committee regarding treatment termination. In his view, further treatment, particularly transfusions, would be futile. When pressed, he explained that further transfusions would be futile because if they "fixed her up," the patient would inevitably be back on the hospital's doorsteps in a few months. He acknowledged that he thought further transfusions would be futile not because they wouldn't work, but because they wouldn't be worth it.

The patient had another perspective and another goal in mind. When asked about her treatment preferences, the patient stated that she wanted to start all over again, that life was worth living, and that she was "kicking the habit."

This case illustrates the nature of the conflict that may exist between patients and physicians over individual judgments of evaluative futility, that is, judgments of whether continued treatment would be worth it. The physician acknowledged that his position in this case did not rest on his clinical judgment about what would be possible medically, but rather on what efforts he thought would be worthwhile. His concern was not that transfusions would not work, but that they would not be worth providing since the patient was an alcoholic.[2] His use of the language of futility demonstrates how personal value judgments and prejudices can be operative under the guise of seemingly objective judgments. It also underscores how some physician judgments of futility may initially be presented as factual when in reality they are clearly evaluative.

The case raises a host of obvious normative questions. Should this physician have been authorized to unilaterally discontinue transfusion therapy on the basis of his evaluative judgment that aggressive treatment of this patient would not be worth it? Are there limits to the kind of evaluative judgments physicians should be authorized to impose? At what point do patient preferences become relevant? Who should be empowered to decide what efforts are worthwhile and what chances for recovery are worth taking? How should the conflict between this physician and patient be adjudicated?

Because the physician viewed the patient's alcoholism as a personal, hopeless, and perhaps deserved problem, he felt less inclined to treat her aggressively. His own prejudices clearly influenced his evaluative judgment of futility. One wonders how frequently evaluative judgments of futility are similarly influenced[3] and what sorts of safeguards would protect patients from discrimination if physician unilateral refusal to provide treatment on the grounds of evaluative futility were sanctioned.

This case demonstrates one possible consequence of granting physicians wide latitude in formulating and imposing their own personal evaluative judgments of futility. But what if physicians were only empowered to impose evaluative judgments that conformed to professional standards and emerging societal norms? Might there be a role for physician unilateral refusal on the grounds of that kind of evaluative futility?

As discussed in Chapter 2, the appropriate treatment of patients in persistent vegetative states is increasingly the subject of critical discussion. An emerging position in the literature, often presented as a reflection of an emerging societal consensus, is that "life" in a persistent vegetative state is not only not worth living, but not worth expending limited public funds and resources to sustain.[4]

Might a physician's agreement with this view be sufficient to justify her unilateral refusal to offer, provide, or continue treatment? Note that the potential conflict here is not just between the individual physician's and the individual patient's personal beliefs about goals worth pursuing. A potential conflict also exists between the individual physician, presumably acting as an agent of her profession and society, and the individual patient, who may disagree with both professional and societal opinion yet not have the power to influence or resist either.

Would physician unilateral refusal to offer, provide, or continue treatment be justified under these circumstances? In other words, if the physician's evaluative judgment of futility is supported by accepted or emerging professional standards or by societal consensus, is her unilateral refusal more justified than if it is based only on her individual personal beliefs and prejudices?

The case that follows provides a forum for considering the proper weight and relevance of professional standards and emerging societal consensus when patients, or the family members that speak for them, disagree.

Case Report #2[5]

A two-year-old boy wandered off into his neighbor's backyard pool during a neighborhood barbecue. He was found some 10 minutes later, lying face-down and pulseless. He was rushed by ambulance to the emergency room where, after defibrillation and drug treatment, his cardiac activity resumed. Two weeks later, the patient was weaned successfully from the ventilator. A trach was performed to facilitate airway maintenance and a g-tube was placed for nutritional support. He was diagnosed as being in a persistent vegetative state.

The patient's parents deeply loved and accepted this child as part of their family and were committed to caring for him at home, along with his 4 other siblings. They understood and accepted his condition, though for the first few months his father seemed hopeful that a cure or miracle would be possible. About 22 months after the accident, the case came to the bioethics committee. The patient had been getting about 4–5 colds a year which often progressed to pneumonia for which he would require short-term hospitalization with ventilatory support and PICU care. Additionally, he had developed severe contractures that required surgery.

The attending physician felt conflicted. He wanted to support the parents' desire for continued maximal care, but he was under intense pressure from the pediatric medical group to refuse to admit the child the next time he presented with pneumonia. His peers cited the issues of futility, professional integrity, and the scarcity of resources. The patient's parents made it very clear that they loved their son, despite his inability to communicate with them. They understood his condition, and accepted that he would never "recover," but they wanted his life preserved.

This case illustrates the nature of the conflict that may exist between patients and physicians when the issue is evaluative futility (that is, whether continued treatment would be worth it), and when emerging professional standards and societal norms might support the physician's decision to deny the treatment. Again, the physician's question about evaluative futility did not rest on his clinical assessment of what would be medically possible for this patient. In fact, the patient's bouts with pneumonia were managed readily in his brief hospital stays, and surgery was a medically viable option for releasing contractures. The nagging question in this physician's mind was whether these medically effective interventions were worth providing for a patient who would never regain consciousness. Appealing to his peers, he would be led to answer the question in the negative. Appealing to the patient's parents, he would be led to answer in the affirmative.

When family values conflict with professional standards and potentially emerging societal norms, which should take precedence? Who should be empowered to select the goals of treatment against which futility should be judged? Should it be the physician group, for whom the goal was restoration of consciousness and function, or the parents, for whom the goal was continued existence? To whom or to what should the patient's physician be committed in cases of conflict? How far should physician authority to impose evaluative judgments extend? What claims, if any, might society have to limit the use of scarce resources for this kind of case?

This case is reminiscent of the *Wanglie* case discussed in Chapter 1.[6] Helga Wanglie's family insisted that she would have thought that life in a persistently vegetative state was worth living. Her physicians thought that continued existence in a persistent vegetative state was not in Helga Wanglie's personal medical interest. Though the court declined to decide which opinion was "right," it did rule that Helga Wanglie's husband of 53 years was the appropriate person to make decisions on her behalf, even in light of the knowledge that her physicians disagreed with his evaluative judgment about her treatment. In this case at least, physician unilateral decision making on the grounds of evaluative futility, even when supported by the local professional community, was rejected.

The third case illustrates the most troubling and problematic aspect of unilateral decision making. If physicians are empowered to unilaterally refuse to offer, provide, or continue treatments on the grounds of evaluative futility, based on their own personal beliefs or sanctioned by professional standards and societal norms, patients might lose any opportunity to make their own goals and evaluative frameworks known. Physicians might thus use unilateral decision making to avoid actual conflicts in values that might otherwise arise in the therapeutic relationship. Rather than involving the patient in a process of shared decision making, in which conflicting values can be discussed and resolved, physicians might be encouraged to make unilateral decisions based on their own particular evaluative judgments or on the evaluative judgments sanctioned by their profession. The patient's evaluative judgments might then be rendered irrelevant. Obviously this shift in physicians's obligations to patients raises a host of ethical concerns.

Case Report #3[7]

A woman from Southeast Asia presented with persistent uncontrollable internal bleeding due to a ruptured large necrotic highly anaplasic cancer of the liver which had previously been shown to be unresponsive to both radiotherapy and chemotherapy. Her physician, aware that no medical interventions would reverse the patient's condition or prevent her death, could have judged any further treatment to be futile and opted for unilateral decision making. Following the popular recommendation, without telling the patient or gaining her consent, and based solely on his medical opinion, he could have written an order to discontinue transfusions and not attempt resuscitation should the patient experience a cardiopulmonary arrest.

Instead, following a protocol he had developed stressing autonomy even when survival was unprecedented, he chose to share all of the available medical information with the patient and solicit her opinion. When confronted with the gravity of her condition, she begged her physician to keep her alive by any means, including transfusions and CPR if necessary. The patient was convinced, based on her cultural and religious belief system, that if she died during that period of time she would inflict a curse upon five generations of her family. Her sole goal and concern was to survive until the moon passed into its next phase.

For this patient, even though transfusions and CPR would not reverse her underlying condition or prevent her ultimate death, they were worth pursuing temporarily. Her goal of short-term survival led her to evaluatively judge the treatments as necessary and worthwhile. Her physician agreed to honor and support her goal.

The power of this case lies in the means by which the physician discovered the central values and goals of the patient: genuine bilateral conversation, not unilateral decision making. Had he unilaterally refused to provide the requested transfusions and CPR on the basis of his judgment of evaluative futility, the physician would have missed the opportunity to discover what was most important to his patient. Had she not been given the opportunity to explain her goals and values, the patient would not have contributed to the calculation of evaluative futility, particularly since her values probably would not have been known or shared by the staff. Because he engaged in direct and bilateral conversation with his patient, the physician was able to discover that the patient had a goal other than mere survival or indefinite prolongation of life. And he was able to discover that he could comfortably assist her efforts in achieving her goals. Unilateral decision making would have denied both patient and physician those opportunities.

In some respects, this case seems highly unusual. The patient's request was not perceived as posing an undue burden on either the physician or society. Her physician was willing to help her achieve a goal that was important to her. Issues of scarcity of resources were not deemed relevant. The moon would pass its required phase in a matter of days, and the blood supply was relatively ample.

But this case is not as unique as it may first appear. In fact, futile support is often continued for patients until out-of-town family members arrive to pay their last respects. In those cases as well, a goal other than reversal of condition or survival is adopted to justify treatment that would otherwise be withdrawn. In cases in which foregoing treatment is an issue, if there is no conversation, there is no opportunity for patient goals to be known, much less honored.

Obviously, conversation alone will not resolve all potential conflicts. Still at issue is the question of how much latitude patients should be given to set the goals of their medical treatment. At what point do a physician's personal values or society's interests enter into the equation? Who should be empowered to judge a treatment to be futile on evaluative grounds? Whose values should ultimately be represented and honored? Should only patients be empowered to make judgments of evaluative futility? Can a physician's evaluative judgment of futility ever be a sufficient justification for unilateral refusal to offer, provide, or continue treatment? At what point can society's interests override the patient's or the physician's?[8] These are the questions to which I now turn.

The Generalization of Expertise Argument

First presented by Veatch in 1973,[9] the generalization of expertise argument provides the most obvious and effective argument against physician unilateral refusal to offer, provide, or continue treatment on the grounds of evaluative futility. In this chapter, I outline the generalization of expertise argument and illustrate its applicability to the discussion of evaluative futility. In Chapter 4, I extend the generalization of expertise argument to show how it can also undermine the normative weight of judgments of factual or physiologic futility.

Because the generalization of expertise argument has been substantially "won," its applicability to the discussion of evaluative futility is intuitively obvious. Much more controversial and novel is the appeal to the argument in my discussion of factual or physiologic futility.

The generalization of expertise argument focusses on the nature of and appropriate limits to knowledge, expertise, and authority. The generalization of expertise argument frames the analysis by asking what kinds of knowledge, expertise, and authority are at stake; whether there are or should be limits to the application of different knowledge, expertise, and authority; and most importantly, whether it is defensible to generalize from one kind of knowledge or expertise to another.

Applied to the futility debate, the generalization of expertise argument would have us begin by asking in what body of knowledge and experience physicians can claim, *qua* physicians, to have particular expertise. Likewise, we would inquire in what body of knowledge and experience patients can claim, *qua* patients, to have particular expertise. The relevance of role-specific expertise is critical. The focus is not on every area of expertise an individual physician or patient might have, but rather on those areas in which they have expertise by virtue of their status as physicians or patients.

As I have established, physicians have traditionally been understood to have expertise in factual medical matters, while patients and their families or other surrogates have been understood to have expertise in the personal normative values that guide their lives and therefore inform their responses to available medical alternatives. The generalization of expertise argument does not challenge seriously this popular conception of role-specific expertise. Rather, it challenges the legitimacy of generalizing or extrapolating from one area of expertise to another. Specifically, the generalization of expertise argument demonstrates that physicians cannot generalize justifiably from their traditionally recognized area of expertise (medical facts) to all other areas of expertise. Though some contributors to the futility debate argue that physicians can and should claim expertise in both the technical and evaluative realms, such a position does not contradict the generalization of expertise argument because physicians' technical expertise itself does not lead automatically to their evaluative expertise.

The idea of role-specific expertise suggests that there are certain realms in which only patients are expert and in which physicians cannot claim legitimately to have expertise by virtue of their role as physicians. For example, physicians, *qua* physicians, cannot claim to be expert in the values that should and do govern medical decision making by patients. Physicians can only articulate what is medically possible, not what is reasonably worth pursuing for a particular patient. Physicians, *qua* physicians, can only know whether transfusions would work for the alcoholic patient, whether short-term ventilatory support and PICU care would work for the pediatric PVS patient, and whether transfusions or CPR would work for the cancer patient. Physicians, *qua* physicians, cannot know whether any of these interventions would be worth it for the particular patients in question.

Succinctly put, because physicians cannot claim to be in an epistemically privileged position when it comes to the personal normative values that inform a patient's decision, they cannot claim to be in a normatively privileged position either.

The generalization of expertise argument takes its bearings from the philosophical distinction between facts and values. All medical treatment decisions have factual and evaluative components. At issue is who has the requisite expertise to determine which facts and which values should govern each decision. In which component of the decision—the factual or the evaluative—can physicians and patients claim exclusive or at least authoritative expertise?[10]

The generalization of expertise argument accepts, in a preliminary way, physicians' claims to expertise about medical facts, but draws the line at their claim to expertise about the personal normative values of particular patients. While physicians may have developed opinions over time about which normative values they think ought to guide decision making, they are not expert in an individual patient's own personal value system. Patients have the most defensible claim of expertise in the personal normative values that guide their lives and therefore their assessment of different treatment possibilities.

Early evidence of the appeal of the generalization of expertise argument can be found in Imbus and Zawacki's study. Though their clinical experience, corroborated by the medical and surgical literature, provided ample evidence that no patients with a specified severity of total body burn had ever survived before, Imbus and Zawacki insisted that such patients be free to make their own decisions about treatment based on their own value systems. As they explained it, the choice about whether to provide or withhold maximal treatment was a moral, not a medical judgment. In other words, medical facts and physician expertise could only go so far. When it came to evaluating the meaning and significance of the facts and choosing a therapeutic option, physicians *qua* physicians could not claim to be in a privileged position. In fact, if a physician's opinion about the therapeutic choice was solicited, Imbus and Zawacki were quick to note that it would be

> merely his personal, inexpert opinion about whether it is better to accept death or fight to make history as the first survivor in such an injury.[11]

Recognizing the difference in physicians' and patients' role-specific expertise, Imbus and Zawacki accordingly structured their approach to burned patients when survival was unprecedented. Because they considered the choice to be moral, not medical, and because they took patient expertise to be central to the task of selecting between conflicting moral values, they focussed on the patient-based principle of autonomy, not on the physician-based principles of beneficence or nonmaleficence.

A similar approach was taken in the landmark case of Karen Ann Quinlan. Again at issue was the question of role-specific expertise. And again, a distinction was made between medical and moral expertise. Karen Ann Quinlan was in what we now call a persistent vegetative state. Though she was not terminally ill, her condition was irreversible. Her physician insisted that all treatment be continued to preserve her life. Her father sought appointment as her guardian in order to request, on her behalf, that "extraordinary heroic" measures be discontinued. A court battle ensued about who had the requisite expertise to decide whether ventilatory support was of sufficient benefit to be continued.

The answer to the question depended on whether the judgment was understood to be factual or evaluative. If Karen Ann Quinlan's physician's testimony that the ventilator provided a benefit was viewed as a strictly factual judgment, then he or the medical profession would be justified in continuing treatment. But, if his judgment of benefit included an evaluative component, then he or the medical profession at large would be unjustified in generalizing from acknowledged technical expertise to unacknowledged evaluative expertise.

Since Karen Ann Quinlan's physician could not claim to have any special expertise in values, he could not claim the right to unilaterally impose his own personal or even his profession's shared values on her. In fact, in granting Mr. Quinlan the right to make medical decisions on behalf of his daughter, the New Jersey Supreme Court confirmed explicitly that the decision about whether to continue ventilatory support was not an exclusively medical one, and hence authority should not reside exclusively with Karen Ann Quinlan's individual physician or the medical profession. The court's decision in favor of Mr. Quinlan affirmed patients' rights of authorship (either in their own voice or through the voice of their surrogates) of the values that govern treatment decisions in their medical care.

In both the Imbus and Zawacki study and the Karen Ann Quinlan case, the choice of therapeutic options was recognized ultimately to be evaluative. In the case of Imbus and Zawacki's burn patients, was aggressive maximal therapy worth it given the reality of unprecedented survival? Or, in the case of Karen Ann Quinlan, was sustained biological life worth it in the absence of any possibility of cognitive sapient existence? The answer to the evaluative question in both of these cases was deemed to be beyond the scope of medical expertise. The medical profession's ascertainment that survival was unprecedented, or that a return to cognitive sapient existence was impossible, went unchallenged. But the medical profession's ability to generalize from that factual expertise to evaluative expertise about the most desirable course of action was flatly rejected.

The legacy of these cases and others like them from the 1970s is the commonly accepted perspective that individual clinicians, and the medical profession at large, can claim legitimately to be experts in describing what *is* the case, but cannot generalize legitimately from that acknowledged expertise to determine what *should* be the case for particular patients.

Commitment to the conclusions of the generalization of expertise argument can be found through much of the contemporary futility literature.

For my purposes, this manifestation of the generalization of expertise argument represents the first level of the futility debate. At this level, the debate addresses the appropriate limit and scope of physician authority in making evaluative judgments. It is at this level that there is the most discussion and consensus. The second level of the debate, which I take up in Chapter 4, concerns the appropriate limit and scope of physician authority in making factual scientific judgments. This area has received much less attention but is equally, if not more, important to a critical analysis of the contemporary trend in favor of physician unilateral refusal on the grounds of futility. The third level of the debate, which I anticipate and address in a preliminary way in Chapter 5, concerns the appropriate limit and scope of patient authority. What can a patient compel a physician to do in cases of conflict over futility?

The generalization of expertise argument laid the groundwork for challenging the authority of physicians to presume evaluative expertise and to impose value judgments on their patients. Though it is rarely acknowledged explicitly, the generalization of expertise argument informs most arguments against physician unilateral refusal on the grounds of strictly evaluative futility.

For example, in early articulations by Youngner and the Hastings Center *Guidelines*, the accepted framework dissuades physicians from generalizing from their acknowledged technical expertise to their unacknowledged evaluative expertise. Even if physicians are in the best position to evaluate hard scientific data regarding the likelihood that a particular treatment will produce certain physiological effects, it is logically impossible for physicians to reach normative conclusions on the basis of those facts alone. They cannot determine, on the sole basis of those facts, which potential benefits of the treatment are worth pursuing for which patients. Because it depends on values and not facts, the latter calculation, unlike the former, resides properly with the patients themselves.

Objections to the Generalization of Expertise Argument

Though the generalization of expertise argument has been regarded traditionally as an accurate account of the appropriate scope and limit of physician authority, several of its key elements have been challenged in ways significant for the futility debate. Scholars such as Edmund D. Pellegrino and David C. Thomasma,[12] Leon R. Kass,[13] Tom Tomlinson and Howard

Brody,[14] Lawrence Schneiderman and Nancy Jecker,[15] and Jecker and Robert Pearlman[16] have challenged the legitimacy of construing the practice of medicine as essentially factual and not evaluative. For these authors, it is an anathema to construe the practice of medicine as anything less than an intrinsically moral enterprise. Accordingly, attempts to wrest from physicians the power to make moral judgments on behalf of patients denies the very expertise and commitments that define the healing profession. Under some interpretations, in fact, the generalization of expertise argument betrays a critical misunderstanding of the enterprise of medicine itself.

Tomlinson and Brody[17] point to the incoherence and implausibility of restricting medical expertise to factual, scientific matters. In their view, medical expertise and practice are linked inextricably to the ability to make and act on judgments of value.

According to Tomlinson and Brody, all medical treatment decisions have an inherent evaluative component about which physicians are qualified uniquely and distinctively to render authoritative opinions. Evaluations of possible medical interventions unavoidably involve evaluative judgments about the likelihood and significance of harms, risks, and benefits. It is a mistake to assume that the factual and evaluative components of medical decision making can be separated neatly.

Jecker and Pearlman sound a similar warning. They note that even seemingly "mundane" decisions about which tests to order, or about how frequently and for what duration they should be performed all involve value judgments, if only about what confidence levels are acceptable. Consistent with Tomlinson and Brody, they argue that,

> [W]e should not attempt in vain to purge medical decision making of any value aspect. Nor should we try to limit physicians' decisional authority to narrow technical issues. We must instead admit that values are inherent in medical choices and integral to the physician's role. Health professionals cannot wash their hands of ethical decision making or attempt to delegate all ethical choices to patients and surrogates.[18]

In addition to rejecting attempts to divorce medical facts from values, this general argument appeals to a broader understanding of the goals of medicine and of the importance of professional integrity. Medicine, the argument goes, is not a value-free enterprise. In fact, it is founded on at least two essential and explicitly stated defining values: the commitment to do good and the commitment to avoid harm. These values, encapsulated in the principles of beneficence and nonmaleficence, form the only basis for the obligation of a physician *qua* physician to enter into a therapeutic relationship with a patient. A physician *qua* physician would not be justified in offering treatments to a patient if the provision of the treatments would violate these foundational principles.

As a matter of professional integrity, the argument continues, physicians have always had, and must continue to have, the authority to control the uses of their skill and knowledge. Otherwise, physicians would be reduced to mere technicians subject to the whims and sometimes irrational fancies of patients.

Replacing the physician-patient relationship with a technician-patient relationship would not only violate physician integrity, it would also fail ultimately to serve genuine patient autonomy. As Tomlinson and Brody explain, the mere act of offering a patient a treatment that the treating physician has deemed futile undermines the patient's ability to make an autonomous choice, because the treatment has already been defined as inconsistent with the patient's interests. To be a member of the healing profession rather than a mere technician is to be committed to making appropriate value judgments in the service of patient interests.

According to Tomlinson and Brody, the issue is not *whether* physicians can or should make value judgments about the worthiness of particular therapeutic options, but rather *which* value judgments physicians may legitimately make in responding to patient requests. Recognizing concerns about the abuse of such power, they propose a model of decision making in which physicians are empowered to employ "reasonable, socially validated value judgments to restrict the alternatives offered to patients."[19] This approach blends a concern for the profession's understanding of its defining values (to do more good than harm) with a recognition of the profession's obligation to be responsive to the larger society in which it practices and from which it derives its social status.

Schneiderman and Jecker take a similar approach, but offer a somewhat different description of the process of social validation. They maintain that physicians have an obligation to make value choices consistent with the patient-centered tradition of medicine.[20] As such they propose not only that physicians be free to withhold or cease futile therapies, but also that they be encouraged and even required to do so. In their schema, it is the responsibility of the medical profession to define the standards of beneficial and

nonbeneficial medical practice and to regulate the scope of individual physician behavior.[21] In so doing the profession rightly claims authorship of the
ethical values and goals that guide the practice of medicine.[22] Though the
public need not passively accept the profession's determinations, the frame
of reference within which critical evaluation takes place is, as I have suggested, somewhat constrained in this approach.

The Argument from Autonomy

Asking not whether, but which value judgments physicians can make in
order to restrict patient access to desired treatment raises obvious concerns
about protecting autonomous patients from unwanted medical paternalism.
From the perspective of patient autonomy, we might even ask not which
value judgments physicians should be entitled to make, or whether they
should make them, but when, i.e., under what circumstances, physicians
should be authorized to substitute their values or their sense of appropriateness for those of their patients.

The argument from autonomy is linked closely to the generalization of
expertise argument. Both focus on the appropriate nature and scope of physician and patient authority. And both address the need to understand the
role-specific perspectives and interests at stake.

The term autonomy has its roots in the Greek words *auto* (meaning self)
and *nomos* (meaning rule, legislation, or determination). Originally the
term *autonomia* described Greek city-states that were independent of outside control. Citizens of these city-states selected their own laws of governance rather than being subjected to laws imposed by an external source.
Self-rule, or autonomy, contrasts with other-rule, or heteronomy. Rather
than being ruled by another, the autonomous individual develops and acts
on her own life plan. Interference with her right to choose her own goals
and ends, or imposition of another's rule instead, subject the autonomous
individual to a heteronomous life. When a physician attempts to substitute
his judgment for his patient's, he is attempting to replace patient autonomy
with heteronomy.

In the clinical context, this is traditionally called the contrast between
patient autonomy and medical paternalism. The overriding of a patient's
autonomous preferences, decisions, or actions out of a concern for the patient's welfare constitutes paternalism. Much has been written about the

different kinds of paternalism and their relative justification in a variety of clinical contexts. To evaluate whether physician unilateral refusal to offer, provide, or continue treatments on the grounds of evaluative futility is an example of paternalism, and to judge whether it is justified, I will review the traditional analysis of paternalism.[23]

The first distinction relevant for our purposes is between limited or weak paternalism and extended or strong paternalism. In limited or weak paternalism, a patient's preferences, decisions, and actions are overridden because there are internal or external constraints on his ability to think and act freely. For example, if a patient is admitted to the emergency room with a drug overdose, or immediately after a near-fatal accident, he may simply not be able to participate in the decisions about his treatment. A physician who treats such a patient against the patient's immediately expressed wishes may claim to be engaging in limited or weak paternalism. A claim of limited or weak paternalism requires diminished patient capacity.

By contrast, in extended or strong paternalism, diminished capacity is not at issue. When physicians intervene and override patient preferences, decisions, and actions in order to protect the patient from harming himself, it is an instance of extended or strong paternalism. Given arguments in support of patient autonomy, this kind of intervention is much harder to justify than limited or weak paternalism.

A second relevant distinction is between soft and hard paternalism. In soft paternalism the values that are used to assess harm and benefit belong to the patient. In hard paternalism the values that are used to assess harm and benefit are alien to, and therefore imposed upon, the patient.

Given this established framework, it is difficult to characterize physician unilateral refusal to offer, provide, or continue treatments on the grounds of evaluative futility as anything other than strong, hard paternalism. Such unilateral refusal is certainly not restricted to patients with diminished capacity, nor does it rely on patient values for guidance. To the contrary, physician unilateral decision making on the basis of futility functions precisely to protect patients from the allegedly bad choices that they might otherwise make, and to substitute for the internal values of the patient the external and alien values of the individual physician or the medical profession. When a physician judges a treatment to be evaluatively futile, she judges it to be not worth providing, despite the patient's capacity or value system. Even though such strong, hard paternalism might be motivated by the best of intentions—the commitment to promote patient welfare or to be a responsible steward of societal resources—it is hard to justify in the face of the argument from autonomy.

It has long been accepted in the clinical context that an essential way of respecting persons is to respect their capacity and right to be autonomous agents with their own independent value systems. Every effort is made, in keeping with the standard of informed consent and informed refusal, to grant competent patients with the requisite decision making capacity the authority to determine what happens to their bodies and lives in accordance with their own value systems.

Granting physicians authority to make unilateral decisions on behalf of patients mistakenly assumes that physicians have the right to rule and legislate on behalf of their otherwise free patients when they disagree with their patients' values or goals. Because the importance of respecting autonomy is accepted so widely, the circumstances in which an individual's autonomy can be overriden have been defined far more narrowly than unilateral refusal on the grounds of evaluative futility would allow.

For example, the authority to override a competent and capable individual's autonomous wishes generally is accepted when those wishes pose an immediate, direct threat of serious harm to a third party. It is much harder to justify interference with an individual's freedom when the motivation is to protect the individual from harming himself, even harder when the values used to justify the intervention are alien to the individual, and harder still when the intervention is made without the patient's knowledge.

One of the most disturbing features of the popular proposals that advocate physician refusal to offer, provide, or continue treatments on the grounds of evaluative futility is that they accept and promote the legitimacy of physician *unilateral* decision making. By definition, "unilateral" implies that patients, even competent patients with the requisite decision making capacity, have no opportunity to participate meaningfully in discussions or decisions about their care. Contrary to the usual respect for patients as autonomous agents, when physicians judge a particular treatment course to be not worth pursuing, patients become subject to the imposition of potentially alien value judgments, in the worst case without their knowledge, participation, or right to refusal, and in the best case, without a genuine opportunity to oppose the physician's decision. Nothing in the therapeutic relationship between physicians and patients supports the deliberate imposition of physicians' own idiosyncratic value judgments (or their profession's values) on patients in this fashion.

The Limits of the Argument from Autonomy

The task of this chapter has been to argue against physician unilateral decision making on the basis of evaluative futility. For that purpose, as an adjunct to the generalization of expertise argument, the argument from autonomy is effective. But it is critical to acknowledge the actual scope and limit of the principle of respect for autonomy. As I have used it thus far, the principle describes a right of noninterference. It delineates a set of limits that are designed to protect an individual from interference and governance by someone or something outside of herself.

To argue that patients have autonomy is to argue that they have the capacity and right to decide for themselves the values and rules that will govern their existence. As such, the argument from autonomy can be marshalled effectively against the proposal of physician unilateral decision making. The argument works because it provides a justification for limiting the power physicians can exercise over patients, specifically the power to make and impose evaluative judgments without their knowledge or consent. If physicians exercised such power over patients, they would violate the capacity and right of patients to self-determination. In essence, granting physicians unilateral decision making power on the basis of evaluative futility would substitute a system of heteronomy for patient autonomy.

While I have appealed to the argument from patient autonomy to reject physician unilateral decision making on the basis of evaluative futility, it is important to recognize that the principle of autonomy itself is insufficient to ground a right of access to treatment. That is, patient autonomy is insufficient to compel a physician to provide treatment she deems futile, and even, perhaps, to compel society to make the treatment available.[24]

The power of the argument from autonomy is limited because it supports a right of noninterference, a negative right, and not a welfare right of entitlement, a positive right. The principle of autonomy does not entitle a patient to receive from physicians anything but the right to noninterference.

Further, the principle of autonomy does not mean that a patient has the capacity and right to decide for others the values and rules that will govern their existence. In that sense, to substitute patient autonomy for physician decision making would be to substitute one system of heteronomy for another. And it is no more justified for a patient to impose his will on a physician than for a physician to impose her will on a patient.

There are limitations to the capacity and right of patients and physicians to decide for themselves the values and rules that will govern their existence. Entering into a therapeutic relationship as a care provider, and entering into a social contract might include the making of certain promises and the acceptance of certain obligations. And, as I suggest in Chapter 5, it might be those very commitments, rather than the principle of autonomy, that ground a right of access to treatment deemed futile by a physician. The physician-patient conflict that has been the focus of my analysis thus far exists within a broader context that must be taken into account, for the details of that context often determine whether or not patients will have a right of access to the treatments they desire.

Concluding Remarks

In this chapter I have considered whether physician unilateral refusal to offer, provide, or continue treatments on the grounds of evaluative futility can be justified. Using the popular approach to futility, I have argued that a physician's judgment that a treatment would be evaluatively futile, or just not worth it, is insufficient to justify unilateral decision making. Appealing to the generalization of expertise argument and to the argument from autonomy, I have suggested that such unilateral refusal extends beyond the acknowledged limit and scope of physician authority to make and impose personal evaluative judgments on patients. The position I have defended is consistent with the popular approach to futility and is generally accepted in the literature. More difficult to prove is the argument I take up in Chapter 4, namely, that physician unilateral refusal on the grounds of physiological or factual futility is similarly unjustified.

THE POWER OF POSITIVIST THINKING[1]
The Problem with Physiologic Futility

Different Approaches to Evaluative and Physiologic Futility

CHAPTER 3 FOCUSSED on the question of whether evaluative futility is a sufficient justification for physician unilateral decision making. Specifically in question was the legitimacy of a physician unilaterally refusing to offer, provide, or continue treatment that was, in her judgment, evaluatively futile. At stake were the issues of who should be empowered to assign meaning and value to medical interventions, and of what should follow normatively once meaning and value are assigned.

In agreement with the approach taken generally in the literature, I have argued against physician unilateral decision making on the basis of evaluative futility. My argument rested on some generally agreed upon substantive assumptions about the nature of evaluative futility judgments (namely, that they are by definition value judgments), and on certain procedural convictions (namely, that when it comes to assigning meaning and value to medical interventions, patients are in a privileged epistemic position and hence their wishes should be given primary consideration.)

Most contributors to the literature answer the "Who should decide?" question differently depending upon the presumed nature of the "what" that is being decided. When the "what" is understood to be substantially evaluative in nature, the literature has tended to favor patients' decision making authority. But when the "what" is understood to be substantially factual in nature, the literature has tended to accede to physicians' decision making authority.

The category of factual or physiologic futility has increasingly been regarded as a useful tool for setting appropriate limits to what patients can expect to receive from their physicians. The popular argument asserts that while patients may be entitled, as an extension of their autonomy, to assign their own value or meaning to particular medical interventions, and to choose their own goals for treatments based on their own life priorities and value systems, physicians can and should constrain the scope of treatment choices made available to patients in meeting those goals.

In other words, patients should only be empowered to select from among those treatment goals their physicians have identified as medically feasible to pursue, and to select from among those means their physicians have identified as effective in achieving the chosen goals.

Physiologic Futility as the Exception to the Rule

Under this popular model, physicians may employ the category of futility to limit the services patients can expect to receive. If a physician deems a treatment to be ineffective or physiologically futile, even if the patient values and specifically requests it, the physician can refuse unilaterally to provide it. Since there is no right to ineffective or physiologically futile treatments, it is argued, physicians should be entitled to make unilateral decisions to not offer, provide, or continue treatments on the basis of physiologic futility.

As Howard Brody explains, while patients may have a critical role in assessing the nature of their medical problems, their role ends when it comes to selecting which treatment options will be offered or made available to them. Those decisions are reserved appropriately for physicians.

> The physician must decide unilaterally whether a treatment possibility comes up to the mark as proper scientific medical practice. . . . The moral value at stake here is the internal integrity and coherence of a professional practice and the maintenance of its internal standards of excellence. . . . Someone who calls himself a physician, but who is constantly willing to compromise on valid modes of treatment in order to satisfy the wishes of the patient, is a fraud. When an intervention is futile, the physician may and indeed should withhold it regardless of the patient's request.[2]

Physiologic futility then becomes a bright line to which physicians can appeal clinically to justify unilateral decision making and to preserve their professional integrity. If the determination of futility turns on the physician's description of the so-called facts, and not on the physician's idiosyncratic values, then the physician, following most of the current literature on futility, would be justified in deciding unilaterally not to offer, provide or continue the treatment in question. Physiologic futility becomes the exception to the rule that otherwise requires physicians to involve patients in the decision making process. As Brody admits,

> The point in determining that intervention X is futile in the situation of patient Y is the implication that the physician may then legitimately withhold X without Y's consent or cooperation.... Thus labeling X as futile effectively renders the decision about whether to administer X an exception to the general duty to respect patient autonomy in therapeutic choices.[3]

Because it is treated routinely as the exception to the rule, physiologic futility deserves especially careful attention. In some respects, it is the hardest and most important test of the general concept of futility. If the concept of futility is to carry the normative moral weight its proponents favor, it must at least be defensible at the level of physiologic futility. In considering the proposed applicability and legitimacy of physiologic futility, we most stringently test the ultimate strength of the concept of futility.

In offering a critical analysis of physiologic futility, my goal is to demonstrate that futility judgments presented as based on indisputable scientific or medical facts have unstated conceptual and evaluative components that significantly undermine their legitimacy as sufficient warrants for physician unilateral decision making. At issue from a clinical and public policy perspective is what should follow normatively from this more complete understanding of the nature of scientific and medical facts. At the very least, I argue, we need a more forthright explication and defense of the various factors that contribute to an understanding of scientific and medical facts, as well as more careful public identification of the points on which we do and do not have consensus, both within and among the scientific community, the medical profession, and the lay population.

I want to be clear at the outset of this portion of the analysis that I am not rejecting the institution of science itself or its applications to clinical medicine. What I suggest, rather, is that we stipulate the existence and availability of scientific and medical data, as well as the system of Western science according to which data are produced, and according to which hypotheses can be tested and conclusions verified. I support this stipulation on pragmatic (rather than metaphysical or epistemological) grounds in order to situate the contemporary futility debate in the context in which it is actually taking place. After all, the futility debate is not about the validity of the enterprise of science itself, but rather about the appropriate interpretation and application of scientific claims to clinical decision making.

Within the parameters of this analysis, Chapter 4 explores the presuppositions underlying the popular position that views factual or physiologic futility as an exception to the rule, and therefore as a sufficient justification for physician unilateral refusal to offer, provide, or continue treatment. Specifically, I locate these presuppositions in a larger philosophical world view—positivism—that is now recognized widely to be fraught with substantial problems. To highlight the problematic features of this world view, I draw on a social constructionist theory of knowledge, which I define and outline below. Though I do not claim social constructionism as a perfect theory, I employ it to draw critical attention to underlying claims rarely addressed explicitly in the contemporary futility debate. Many of the questions that will undoubtedly be raised in response to this analysis are, I would argue, the very questions to which we should be turning our collective attention, for they point the way to the real and unresolved issues at stake in the futility debate.

The Fact-Value Distinction Revisited

The philosophical world view in which the popular stance on physiologic futility is rooted has at its core a number of faulty presuppositions. I will first examine what I take to be three of the most influential presuppositions, and then outline the problems inherent in any position that rests on them.

We Can Know the Truth

The first, and perhaps most important presupposition in the philosophical world view underlying the popular stance on futility concerns what we can know and how we come to know it. The presumption has roots in the philosophical legacy of positivism.[4] Though largely discredited as a viable philosophical school of thought, traces of positivism can still be found throughout the futility debate, especially in the popular treatment of physiologic futility.

A central tenet of positivism that has been especially influential in the formulation of positions on physiologic futility is the conviction that there exists an objective reality that is accessible to us in a direct and unmediated way. Under this model, what we know in certain realms is considered to be a pure reflection of that objective reality.

The notion of reflection or correspondence is key here. Our knowledge reflects and corresponds exactly to what actually "is." Accordingly, that which we can know to be the case factually reflects and corresponds to that which is there to be known.[5] The source of our knowledge, then, is the reality and truth that exists outside of us.

Against this backdrop of orienting beliefs, facts are accorded a privileged status. By virtue of their reflection of and correspondence to the truth, facts are characterized as pure, objective, unbiased, and, most importantly for our investigation, value-free. Conversely, because they are understood to come not from some ultimate reality outside of us, but rather from some idiosyncratic, subjective, context-dependent reality inside of us, values are construed as unreliable and inappropriate indicators of the objective truth. At best, our values reflect each of our subjective realities, but fail to reflect or correspond to the objective truth.

To the extent that facts are accorded a privileged status with respect to values in the futility debate, the presumption that genuine knowledge reflects and corresponds to some objective reality and truth retains its stronghold.

The Autonomy of Knowledge Credo

The second and related presupposition in the philosophical world view that has shaped the popular stance on futility is the long-standing belief that knowledge can be autonomous and pure. This has traditionally been called the autonomy of knowledge credo. If we recall the original meaning of autonomy as self-governing, we can grasp the credo's picture of knowledge as insulated from or immune to outside control and influence.

Under this model, the pursuit of knowledge must necessarily be value-free, objective, dispassionate, context-independent, and free from outside controlling influences. The seeker of knowledge must be similarly unfettered. In other words, the particular values, subjective concerns, interests, and needs of the seeker of knowledge, as well as the social, political, personal, economic, and other contexts in which she seeks knowledge, must all be non-controlling and non-governing. If they were controlling or governing, that would represent heteronomy over knowledge, or, in other words, the susceptibility of knowledge-seeking to values, subjectivity, context, and the like.

Another way of saying that knowledge is autonomous is to say that the identity of the seeker of knowledge and the context of the pursuit make no difference.

Using the Scientific Method Will Lead Us to the Truth

The final and related presupposition underlying the popular treatment of futility is that the scientific method gives us the pure and unbiased access to reality and truth that makes knowledge autonomous and therefore objective and reliable.

The idea is that we can trust in the truths uncovered by science precisely because they are uncovered by a method and general approach that is itself clearly distinct from and independent of context and other biasing and controlling influences. In this view, science generally, and the scientific method specifically, function "above the fray."

To appreciate the powerful appeal of the scientific method, one must understand the difference this view posits between the constitutive and contextual values of science.[6] According to this approach, the constitutive values of science govern the practice of science, regardless of the subject of scientific inquiry, and regardless of the context in which the inquiry is situated. The constitutive values do not just guide scientific practice; they *are* scientific practice. The constitutive values of science distinguish it from other modes of inquiry.

For example, simplicity, replicability, accuracy, predictability, and consistency have all been suggested as values that constitute and guide scientific research. Along with other values, they inform scientists' understanding of what constitutes good scientific practice, a good explanation, a justified conclusion, and so on. Most importantly, they keep scientific practice pure and free from outside controlling influences.

Contextual values, on the other hand, have to do with the context in which science is actually practiced. These values, which can be social, political, personal, or economic have the potential to taint or control the purity of scientific pursuits.

In fact, according to this traditional view of science, if the scientific method is followed faithfully, the only possible source of interference or bias rests with the contextual values that shape the environment within which science is practiced, and not with the values that constitute and guide the actual practice of science itself. "Bad science" is "bad" because contextual values have been allowed to taint or control an otherwise inherently pure and unbiased pursuit of scientific knowledge.

It is important to note that the philosophical world view undergirding the popular treatment of futility conceives of science's constitutive values as distinct from and independent of its contextual values.

In other words, the values that guide scientific practice are autonomous and pure, thereby ensuring that the products of scientific investigation are purely objective and factual. Scientifically discovered truths are free from the control and influence of the values of the investigating scientist or physician, as well as from the contextual values surrounding the investigation itself.

In the futility debate this line of thinking makes an exception for physiologic futility precisely because it presumes that physiologic futility, unlike evaluative futility, is a true objective fact that is discoverable and provable scientifically. In somewhat simplistic terms, physiologic futility is the exception because it is factually, not evaluatively, based.

According to the most popular treatment of futility, the category of physiologic futility describes, in pure, objective, truthful terms what actually *is* the case. The category of evaluative futility, on the other hand, describes what interested parties think *ought* be the case. Only the former is presumed to be sufficient to justify unilateral decision making.

In light of these beliefs, it is not surprising that empirical studies, prognostic tools, and outcome data are marshalled to support arguments in favor of physician unilateral refusal on the grounds of physiologic futility. If a given treatment can be discovered and scientifically "proven" to be ineffective, then it would qualify under the exception and could serve as a justifiable ground for physician unilateral decision making. A review of the recent futility literature provides evidence of the appeal and influence of scientific approaches to quantifying and "proving" physiologic futility.[7]

As we shall now see, science's constitutive and contextual values are not as clearly distinguishable as the popular approach would have us believe. Though the practice of making an exception for physiologic futility on the grounds that it is discoverable scientifically (and therefore objectively) has popular appeal, its underlying presumptions are open to a series of damaging criticisms.

A Social Constructionist Critique

The preceding three foundational presuppositions together constitute a broad philosophical world view that has been enormously influential in the contemporary futility debate. For the purposes of analysis, I have artificially separated the different presuppositions and described them individually. Now, having outlined each of the presuppositions, I will treat them as they actually operate in the futility debate—that is, as integrated components of a broader philosophical world view. I will describe the substantial problems and outline some of the most damaging criticisms of this world view. The problems and criticisms I describe, although presented individually, apply to the philosophical world view as a whole, not to any one presumption.

The most significant problems inherent in the world view include, but are not limited to, the problems of objectivity, value neutrality, method, interpretation, uncertainty, and mistakes. For purposes of clarity, I will discuss each of the problems in turn.

The Problem of Objectivity

One extension of the idea that we can have direct unmediated access to reality is the notion that if we follow the correct method, our resulting knowledge will be somehow purely objective, and therefore will be appropriately privileged. To say that such knowledge is objective in this traditional sense is to say that it reflects a grasp of what actually exists, independent of whatever subjective wishes, biases, distortions, or self-interested motives we might have as seekers of knowledge.

A commitment to objectivity is, most simply put, a commitment to let our beliefs be determined by the impartial, nonarbitrary, verifiable "facts." It is a commitment based on the belief that if we all pursue our inquiries in an objective fashion, keeping a check on potentially tainting subjective influences, then we will all inevitably come to the same conclusions. If we emulate the qualities we attribute to objectivity, such as disinterestedness, detachment, dispassionateness, and universality, the results of our inquiry will embody those characteristics.[8] We will come to the same conclusions ultimately because they will reflect and correspond to a reality that exists beyond all of our individual selves.

Allan Megill puts it nicely in *Rethinking Objectivity* when he says this kind of objectivity

> aspires to a knowledge so faithful to reality as to suffer no distortion, and toward which all inquirers of good will are destined to converge.[9]

This conception of objectivity is not without problems. The most damaging criticism can be located in the social constructionist theory of knowledge. This antipositivist theory has been embraced in a number of disciplines, including the history, philosophy, and sociology of science;[10] literary criticism;[11] and feminist criticism.[12]

For each of these disciplines, the antipositivist turn has meant a focus on particular sources of knowledge and truth. In the history, philosophy, and sociology of science, the focus has been on the contextual circumstances and theoretical commitments that influence the pursuit of knowledge; in literary criticism, on textuality as the condition of all knowledge; in feminist criticism, on context, situatedness, and power.

As we will see, the social constructionist theory of knowledge poses serious challenges to the popular stance of privileging judgments of physiologic futility. Social constructionists would understand judgments of physiologic futility to reflect not some ultimate indisputable objective reality, but rather the broad context in which futility judgments are formulated and defended. As I have indicated, I find this theory and orientation, while not perfect, the most promising and persuasive in criticizing the popular treatment of futility.

An obvious concern raised by a social constructionist theory of knowledge is that it seems to obviate the possibility that there is an "out there" there, i.e., something real that exists outside of ourselves. It is possible, however, to use a social constructionist theory of knowledge to critique the practice of making an exception of physiologic futility, without taking a position on whether an objective reality actually exists. It is sufficient for my purposes to note that whether or not such a reality actually exists, we can never have unmediated access to it. In other words, our access to that reality will always be limited by the lenses through which we see it, conceptualize it, and relate to it. That such lenses are operative I take as a given. Which lenses in particular are operative and whether they are identified explicitly are the more interesting questions to ask. As I argue in Chapter 5, naming and owning of the lenses, and subjecting them to public endorsement or rejection will be the first step in resolving the problem of futility.

To fully appreciate the impact a social constructionist approach would have on the contemporary futility debate, we must consider its orienting methodological concerns. Early thinkers in the philosophy of science, such as Ludwik Fleck[13] and Thomas Kuhn,[14] provided some of the first articulations of a social constructionist theory of knowledge. They stressed the importance of examining the underlying social and cultural forces that lead to the development of scientific facts and understandings. For both Fleck and Kuhn, and others who followed their lead,

> Facts are not phenomena revealed but ideas that are constructed as much socially as intellectually and that depend on the dominant point of view of the scientific community.[15]

At its heart, the social constructionist model rejects the positivist understanding of knowledge and truth as reflecting and corresponding to some objective reality. In its place it posits a model of dynamic interplay among who we are; how, and at what point in time we are situated; and what we know. The source of our knowledge rests substantially and unavoidably within and around us as subjective selves.

The suggestion that facts are not revealed phenomena but constructed ideas raises obvious questions about how ideas are constructed, specifically who constructs them and on what basis. The social constructionist tradition frames these questions as central. Scientific hypotheses, research agendas, theories, representations, explanations, and resultant fact-statements are not reflections of objective reality, but rather products of the theoretical, political, economic, cultural, and social milieu in which they are located. Thus the sharp distinction between constitutive and contextual values cannot be sustained.

In this view, science is understood to be, most fundamentally, a social practice, with its own specific rules and orientations to problems, its own biases about the kinds of knowledge worth pursuing, and its own particular relation to the world around it. As a social practice, science initiates its practitioners into particular theoretical traditions complete with stock sets of orienting questions, foundational tenets, and accepted research and experimental techniques. The discipline is designed to build upon itself, with new understandings evolving against the backdrop of prior collective practice that is situated in a broader societal context, replete with all of its contributing influences.

Hence scientific knowledge has its source not in direct unmediated contact with some objective reality, but in the variety of influences—personal, professional, and societal—that converge to create our understanding of the "truth." At its heart, the social constructionist approach represents a rejection of the autonomy of knowledge credo that has been so influential in the futility debate. It is impossible for science to be totally insulated from or immune to outside control or influence precisely because such a view from nowhere[16] is unattainable. The pursuit of knowledge, including knowledge about what treatments are physiologically futile, can never be purely objective and context-independent.

According to this understanding, even at the level of theory it is impossible to begin from a purely unfettered perspective. In fact, there is a "theory-ladenness" to our understanding of reality that necessarily guides and limits what we set out to observe or measure and what we ultimately come to know.

In the positivist model, our observations come first; only after our indirect, mediated contact with the objective reality do we explain it with theories. In the antipositivist model, "theory has epistemological priority over observation."[17] That is to say, there is no unmediated direct pure access to an objective true reality. Everything we see or know is mediated through our own particular lenses. Accordingly, antipostivists urge us to give up our obsession with truth and representation and focus instead on the task of deconstructing the nature and source of knowledge claims. Contrary to traditional positivist epistemology, who the knowers are and how they are situated become the central epistemological preoccupations. As Lorraine Code explains:

> Once one takes seriously the contention . . . that knowledge is a construct produced by cognitive agents within diverse social practices and positions of differing power and privilege, . . . factors pertinent to the circumstances of the subjects-as-knowers will move to a pivotal place.[18]

In this respect the social constructionist theory of knowledge can offer corrections to prior epistemological approaches that mistakenly accepted as given the "truths" presented by certain privileged members of society. Along those lines, feminists and other theorists have extended social constructionist methodology to uncover ideological biases that have been subsumed systematically under claims to objective factual knowledge.

Some feminist scholars go so far as to argue that accepting traditional conceptions of objectivity may serve only to perpetuate the values held most dearly by the dominant members of society and to hide what should be recognized as clear manifestations of power differentials. According to this interpretation, traditional objectivity and its context-independent and theory/value-neutral stance are driven by distinctive ideological concerns. For some feminist epistemologists,

Scientifically accredited facts are not the hard, incontrovertible, immutable givens they are purported to be, but rather ideological fragments.[19]

It would be interesting for our purposes to consider what and whose interests are similarly served by positing the objective facticity of physiologic futility claims. An object worthy of inquiry at this historical juncture in the evolution of health care is the use of the concept of futility by the medical profession, managed care delivery systems, and governmental funding agencies. Who finds the concept of physiologic futility appealing and why? What do they stand to gain from widespread implementation of the concept?

The Problem of Value Neutrality

The popular practice of making an exception of physiologic futility has been bolstered by the contention that judgments of physiologic futility are purely factual claims devoid of any evaluative content. This understanding of physiologic futility, and the sharp distinction that it presumes to exist between facts and values, has its roots in an older, but now generally repudiated, conception of science.

As our discussion of the problem of objectivity has already suggested, the older conception evidences a fundamental misunderstanding of the actual nature and source of factual knowledge claims. As has been demonstrated, so-called purely factual claims of objective knowledge are socially constructed, and hence beholden, to various degrees, to the theoretical, political, economic, cultural, and social milieu from which they are derived. They are also influenced by the values and theories embedded in that milieu, and by the values and theories held, consciously or unconsciously, by the individual seeking (and brokering) knowledge in that milieu.

The seeker of knowledge and the context of the search matter fundamentally in this model, for they unavoidably influence, albeit to varying degrees, all resultant knowledge claims. Accordingly, the pursuit of knowledge, either general or scientific, can never be completely objective or value-free. The claim that there can be no value-free science has gained widespread acceptance. But the relevance of this claim to the futility debate has received little attention.[20]

To address that concern, I will examine more closely how the values embedded in the social context of knowledge-seeking, and held by the knowledge seeker, are instrumental in the construction of knowledge, and hence in the determination of what is factual.

One classic way of understanding the relationship among context, knowledge seeker, and resulting knowledge claims in science is what Helen E. Longino calls the externality model.[21] Under this model, the values that influence the practice of science are understood to be fundamentally external to the practice itself. That is, while the points of contact between science and the values of the complex milieu in which it is practiced may determine the focus and scope of scientific inquiry, they do not influence the actual conclusions scientists draw, or the explanations of phenomena they provide.

The context in which science is practiced may influence the determination of which questions to ask, which areas of research to pursue, which kinds of research to fund, et cetera, but it does not influence the actual practice of science itself. At the level of practice, the externality model assumes, science can remain autonomous.

The externality model relies heavily on the sustainability of this distinction between the contextual and constitutive values of science. The distinction has long been thought to ensure the integrity of the practice of science itself.[22] In fact, any indication of the influence of contextual values has traditionally been seen as evidence that the science in question is impure or "bad."

But critics have argued that constitutive and contextual values are not as neatly distinguishable as the externality model would suggest. Increasingly, examples have been offered of the creep of contextual values into the realm of constitutive values, and into the construction of scientific knowledge.

In *Science as Social Knowledge*, Longino offers a critique of the externality model by discussing ways in which apparently contextual values can shape the construction of scientific knowledge at the level of practices, questions, data, specific assumptions, and even general assumptions.[23] Examples of this dynamic can also be found in other sources[24] that pose useful analogues to the popular discussion of futility.

Carol Korenbrot's analysis of the early development of oral contraceptives offers an interesting case in point.[25] Korenbrot found that the selection of risks to be measured in research on contraceptives was clearly a function of the extrascientific values of those doing the testing. In other words, who the knowledge seeker was and what his values were influenced the nature of the knowledge that was ultimately produced.

Korenbrot takes Gregory Pincus to be one of the key seekers of knowledge about contraceptives in the 1960s. Her review of *The Control of Fertil-*

ity[26] demonstrates Pincus's overwhelming orienting concern with the value of population control. Birth control was to be used as a weapon against what the author perceived as unchecked and therefore dangerous population growth. Korenbrot contends that Pincus's explicit interest in finding an effective means of controlling population growth strongly influenced his approach to testing the drug Enovid, and led him to place greater emphasis on Enovid's positive effects than on its negative ones. The fact that he was one of the primary scientists involved in developing the drug is also cited as noteworthy.

Korenbrot presents her study of Pincus as an example of how extrascientific concerns can influence the way scientific research is conducted. For our purposes, it stands as an example of how operative contextual values can function, not externally to the constitutive values of science, but in fact as an integral part of their expression in practice. Korenbrot demonstrates how the process of research topic selection, design, and focus, as well as the process of data interpretation and, significantly, the research conclusions themselves, were all influenced by operative contextual values.

D. Alan Shewmon's work on the determination of brain death offers another example of the role of values in constituting the scientific approach to a difficult clinical problem.[27] Shewmon's concern is with the influence of clinicians' notions of acceptable error on their preferred method of determining death. He points out rightly that the tests and criteria employed, as well as the guidelines clinicians support, are determined fundamentally by the kind of error they place the highest value on avoiding.

Whether one most fears mistakenly declaring a live patient dead or disrespectfully treating a cadaver determines the kind of clinical guidelines one will support and the level of certainty one will require in making the determination of death.[28] Accordingly, Shewmon's acknowledged desire to ensure that no live person will ever be diagnosed mistakenly as dead leads him to insist upon a higher degree of certainty than others with different orienting concerns might adopt. Along the same lines, while some neurologists believe that we can measure accurately the irreversible loss of brain function, other neurologists, appealing to different standards of evidence, are not convinced that we can.

It is important for our purposes to recognize that in either case, the underlying concerns, be they evaluative or metaphysical, actually determine what clinical signs are tested for and measured, what test results are weighted more heavily, what level of certainty is deemed sufficient, and what clinical conclusions are drawn. Hence even the scientifically based determination of death is neither context-free nor value-neutral.

Yet another example worth considering comes from the new and increasingly popular field of outcomes research. Because outcomes studies have been marshalled frequently to support claims that particular treatments are futile, it is enlightening to trace the way in which values have influenced the construction of knowledge in that arena as well.

In a telling case in point, the federal Agency for Health Care Policy and Research sponsored three doctors from Harvard Medical School's health care policy department to study the effectiveness of invasive procedures after heart attacks. Based on their analysis of data on 200,000 elderly patients, the researchers concluded that invasive treatments after heart attacks, such as bypass operations and catheterizations, could be reduced by over 25% without increasing mortality.[29] In reporting their study results, the researchers suggested that tremendous savings in communal resources could be achieved annually by offering fewer invasive treatments and focussing attention instead on early noninvasive interventions.

In a striking display of how orienting values and concerns influence research topic selection, design, and focus, as well as the process of data interpretation and, significantly, research conclusions, the researchers note that their study did not measure or address other benefits that could come from the invasive procedures, like improved quality of life due to the therapies' relief of chronic angina or chest pain.

Their focus on long-term survival and their concern for the rising cost of treating heart attacks (a concern shared by their sponsoring agency) led them not only to interpret the data differently, but also to draw different descriptive and normative conclusions than they would have with a different frame of reference, such as quality of life, in mind.

Howard Brody reveals how prior value commitments may likewise influence medical determinations of physiologic futility. First he notes that "[t]he physiologic definition [of futility] appears to offer a value-free judgment, but this turns out to be a false appearance."[30] He then goes on to explain that a treatment is judged to be physiologically futile not because it fails to produce any physiologic effect, but rather because it fails to produce a physiologic effect that is deemed worthy of desire by the individual measuring the effect.

This raises the obvious question of who should determine which effects are worthy of desire. For some proponents of futility, it should clearly be up to physicians to determine the worthiness of desires. Recognition that even judgments of physiologic futility have an evaluative component merely strengthens their resolve to ensure that physicians be empowered to make the right value judgments on behalf of patients. Schneiderman, Jecker, and Jonsen explain, for example:

> Contrary to the assertion that physiologic futility is value-free, we argue that it entails a value choice. Specifically, it assumes that the goals of medicine are to preserve organ function, body parts, and physiologic activity— an assumption that, in our estimation, departs dramatically from the patient-centered goals of medicine.[31]

For them, acceding to patient wishes to provide physiologically futile treatments entails not only a clear value choice, but the wrong value choice, a choice the medical profession has an obligation to correct.

All of these examples illustrate the degree to which values unavoidably, systematically, and in some instances deliberately influence science, and, by extension, clinical medicine at the theoretical, methodological, and practical levels. It is impossible to strip underlying values and perspectives from the context in which scientific and clinical knowledge is sought or from the seekers of that knowledge. There is no value-neutral perspective from which to engage in the enterprise. There are no knowledge claims that can be presented as completely value-neutral. For some of the strongest proponents of futility, it is even inappropriate to strive for such neutrality. In light of this reality, the question becomes: Which and whose values are operative and with what justification?

The Problem of Method

Traditionally science has tried to deflect the criticisms outlined above by insisting that its method, if used properly, assures the reliability and objectivity of research results. The traditional conception of the enterprise of science locates the distinctiveness and authority of science in its method.

Relying on nonarbitrary criteria for formulating, embracing, and discarding explanatory hypotheses and theories; organizing and managing data collection; subjecting experimental findings to rigorous requirements of verification and nonfalsifiability, including an insistence upon replicability of results; and seeking an unbiased understanding of the universe, with all its causal and explanatory relations, are all defining features of the scientific method.

The obvious critical response has been to argue that methodological constraints are insufficient. The constraints themselves—their particular construction, their perceived need, and the problems they are designed to address—are influenced inevitably by the broader context in which they are situated. Furthermore, the methods used by science are discipline-specific and closely linked to the particular phenomena that are under study.[32] No overarching, universal, singular scientific method exists; methods of scientific inquiry are constructed by particular individuals who are seeking particular kinds of knowledge about particular objects or relations.

From this critical vantage point, it is hard to imagine a method that would guard adequately against the problems of objectivity and value neutrality. An inquiry into the related problems of interpretation, uncertainty, and mistakes further undercuts the power of so-called fact claims that have been derived scientifically.

The Problem of Interpretation

The problem of interpretation is related to the difficulty of distinguishing what we bring to the process of observation from what we end up observing. What we bring to the process can be as powerful and particular as our prior experience and history, our language, our bodies, our relative power, our stock orienting questions, our strongly held beliefs, and our underlying theories and conceptual frameworks.[33] All that we bring to the task of investigation can influence what we expect to find, where we look, how we investigate, what we pay attention to, what we ignore, what we count as supporting evidence, et cetera. In other words, we can never conduct an investigation from the perspective of a blank slate on which the object "out there" will make its pure impression. Rather, we refract all of our experiences through the distinctive lenses we bring to the process. And our interpretations are governed accordingly.

Francis Bacon bemoaned the ways in which the mind uses its already existing theoretical lens to make sense of new experiences. He explained,

> The human understanding when it has once adopted an opinion (either as being the received opinion or as being agreeable to itself) draws all things else to support and agree with it.[34]

Bacon's comments are far more than a description of the effects of obvious bias. They extend to a recognition of the subtle ways in which our minds frame and test new experiences in terms of opinions and theories we have already accepted.

Helen Longino adds a twist to this point by suggesting that scientific reasoning by its very nature is particularly susceptible to the influence of pre-existing frames of reference that she calls background beliefs. She asserts,

> How one determines evidential relevance, why one takes some state of af-
> fairs as evidence for one hypothesis rather than for another, depends on
> one's other beliefs, which we can call background beliefs or assumptions.[35]

According to Longino, scientific reasoning is evidential, evidential reasoning is necessarily context-dependent, and background beliefs provide the context that enables us to reason scientifically. They are what allow us to posit connections between observed phenomena, to take experimental results as evidence for hypotheses, and to draw scientific conclusions.

Longino offers several helpful examples to illustrate how background beliefs operate. To explain that the same state of affairs can be taken as evidence for conflicting hypotheses, she describes a young child with red spots on her stomach. Depending upon one's background beliefs, one might take the spots as evidence that the child has measles, or as evidence that she has some kind of gastric disorder. At stake in the evidential reasoning in this case is the meaning accorded in one's belief system to red spots on the stomach.

Red spots on the stomach, or any other phenomenon, do not, Longino says, "carry labels indicating that for which they are evidence."[36] Background beliefs fill in that missing gap in the reasoning. And as the observers and interpreters, we bring the background beliefs into the process. So what we come to know and believe is determined at least in part by what we bring to the process of knowing and believing itself.

In another example, Longino illustrates how different background beliefs can lead us to pick as evidentially relevant different aspects of the same state of affairs. She describes a situation in which two men enter a home and conclude, upon seeing a gray hat on the banister, that Nick is inside.

When asked why they think Nick is in the house, the men offer different reasons. One man explains that Nick is the only person he knows who owns a hat just that shade of gray. The other man explains that Nick is the only person he knows who always throws his hat on the banister in just that way. Though their different beliefs lead them to take different aspects of the hat to be relevant—one its color, the other its location—the two men draw the same conclusion.

What Longino hopes to illustrate by these different examples is that

> [A] given state of affairs can be taken as evidence for quite different and even conflicting hypotheses given appropriately conflicting background beliefs. Similarly, different aspects of one state of affairs can be taken as evidence for the same hypothesis in light of different background beliefs.[37]

Longino also uses the concept of background beliefs to explain how two experimenters working in different theoretical frameworks can come to different conclusions based on the same observations.[38] Differing background beliefs lead them to attend to different aspects of what they are observing and subsequently to draw different conclusions.

Relating these insights to the futility debate, one finds a new way of deconstructing the arguments supporting the exception for physiologic futility. Schneiderman, Jecker, and Jonsen provide a nice example.[39] Because of their background beliefs, these authors choose futility as the interpretation for the observation that a given intervention has failed to "work" in the last 100 cases.

We can immediately recognize that their chosen interpretation of futility might be based on their underlying background beliefs, such as what it means to "work," or, in their language, to "benefit the patient" sufficiently, as well as on how they measure the achievement of these goals. If "futility" is not the only interpretation one might draw from such evidence, the standing accorded to a judgment of physiologic futility as an indisputably accurate representation of the objective truth must be called into question. Schneiderman, Jecker, and Jonsen clarify in their later work that they selected a 1 in 100 chance not to give the illusion of objectivity, but to serve as a reasonable standard based in common sense.[40] The question of course is whether patients in general share their sense of reasonability or the background beliefs from which it is derived.

Using 100 failed past cases as the requisite and sufficient evidence for quantitative, or physiologic, futility employs certain values that may not enjoy widespread support. Some patients or physicians will interpret a 1 in 101 chance (the odds for the next patient) to be worth it. Others will feel confident of their ability to beat the odds, or will insist that they at least be given the opportunity to do so. The Schneiderman, Jecker, Jonsen approach is problematic because the authors have picked a p value (the probability that the findings observed could have happened by chance alone) based on their own background beliefs or the background beliefs of the scientific community without seeking public endorsement of the resultant standard.

Their decision becomes further suspect when one realizes that the odds of the 101st case turning out differently than the prior 100 are calculated differently depending on the underlying statistical theories used. There are a number of fundamentally different ways of statistically interpreting the same data, and different approaches (for example, Baysian or non-Baysian) yield different conclusions.[41]

So the Schneiderman, Jecker, Jonsen approach illustrates the degree to which one's conceptual framework, including one's theoretical commitments and background beliefs, function as a filter through which observations are interpreted and conclusions are drawn. The possibility of reasoning in a purely objective, neutral, value-free, context-independent fashion is again shown to be an unachievable fantasy. As this critical analysis proceeds, it becomes less philosophically tenable to make an exception of physiologic futility in virtue of its privileged status as a "fact," as the popular debate would urge us to do.

It is critical to note here that I am not suggesting that public policy and clinical standards should never be influenced by values. In fact, I am asserting exactly the opposite. We must stop pretending that our underlying values, perspectives, and place in the world do not influence the judgments we make and the positions for which we argue. I am calling for a more honest disclosure of and subsequent defense of these influences with respect to judgments of futility. And I am calling for a process by which values and other influences can be subject to public scrutiny and subsequent endorsement or rejection. Couching judgments of futility in the language of scientific certainty conceals the need for this more careful examination. Two further problems undercut the practice of privileging judgments of physiologic or "factual" futility: the related problems of uncertainty and mistakes.

The Problem of Uncertainty

The problem of uncertainty permeates the practice of clinical medicine. Despite the vast statistical data at their disposal, and despite their developed clinical acumen, when confronted with particular patients, physicians are capable only of making assertions of high probability, not logical certainty. That is the best that science and medicine can ever hope to offer.

There is an inherent and obvious element of uncertainty in clinical medicine. How a particular patient will respond biochemically, physiologically, psychologically, and spiritually to her condition; how particular medications and interventions will affect her body's ability to heal; and how her affect and will to survive will influence her condition are all questions to which there are inevitably uncertain answers.

Despite all we know scientifically and medically, a vast area of knowledge and understanding remains a mystery to us, especially with respect to particular patients. In part this is what makes medicine not just a science, but also and unequivocally an art.

Interestingly, despite the uncertainty at the heart of the art of medicine, judgments of physiologic futility are deceptively, or at best mistakenly, presented as indisputable "facts" and therefore reliable representations of the absolute truth. In the end, the cloak of certainty around the diagnostic and prognostic assessments that ground judgments of physiologic futility becomes an unattainable illusion.

The issue then becomes what degree of imperfect certainty, if any, is acceptable for grounding a judgment of physiologic futility. Once we accept that we cannot have absolute predictive certainty, might any degree of certainty be sufficient? The question, while absolutely appropriate, reveals the recurrent problem behind treating physiologic futility as an exception. In fact, as discussed earlier, the selection of an acceptable level of certainty itself can only be made on evaluative, not factual grounds. That is to say, judgments of physiologic futility necessarily have at their base an evaluative judgment, if only a judgment about the degree of certainty one finds acceptable and unacceptable. And again, the question is whose values should be determinative in selecting acceptable degrees of certainty?

The Problem of Mistakes

Finally, it is an undisputed truth in medicine that physicians not only lack the power to predict perfectly and accurately specific patients' particular courses, but they also, despite their best intentions, make errors. In fact, an entire field has developed around the study of how mistakes are made and handled in clinical medicine. In *The Unity of Mistakes: A Phenomenological Interpretation of Medical Work*,[42] Marianne A. Paget defended the thesis that clinical medicine is an inherently error-ridden activity. She argued that, because medicine is intrinsically experimental, uncertain, and prone to error, mistakes are unavoidable. Charles L. Bosk[43] and Marcia Millman[44] take a similar approach in their respective classic and chilling accounts of how and why mistakes occur, and how they are systematically managed by the modern medical establishment.

The fact that errors are routinely and unavoidably made in medicine, at the level of both scientific theory and clinical practice, should give us pause when we consider the certainty with which judgments of physiologic futility are presented typically. Examples of judgments of futility ultimately being proved wrong can be found readily at both the theoretical and practical levels. Incomplete or faulty explanatory theories, as well as misdiagnoses or misprognoses are well chronicled in the history of medicine. I offer a few examples here to illustrate the degree to which judgments presented as factually and scientifically correct, may be shown to be false.

At the level of scientific theory, the recent debate over the actual cause of and appropriate treatment for peptic ulcers stands as an important example. Though peptic ulcers were traditionally described as a chronic illness exacerbated by stress and diet, new research has confirmed instead that peptic ulcers have a bacterial cause. The clinical applications of this scientific error are astounding. No matter how many drugs a peptic ulcer patient takes to reduce the production or presence of stomach acid, no matter how much rest he gets, and no matter how bland a diet he follows, his ulcer will never be cured. It is now understood that only antimicrobial drugs offer the desired cure.

This dramatic change in understanding was bolstered by a February 1994 recommendation in favor of antimicrobial drugs as the treatment of choice for peptic ulcers made by an independent panel convened by the National Institutes of Health.[45] In fact, the discovery of the bacterium H. Pylori's causal role in peptic ulcer had been made eleven years earlier by two Australian scientists whose reports were not taken seriously.[46] It took the established medical community over a decade to assimilate and validate the provocative findings.

Prior to the discovery of H. Pylori's causal role in peptic ulcers, scientists and clinicians alike would have considered it "futile" in the physiologic or factual sense to treat peptic ulcers with antibiotics. In fact, had a patient requested antibiotics on the basis of the early reports, a physician would likely have considered such treatment physiologically futile. Now, with respect to the goal of cure, scientists and clinicians alike would consider it "futile" in the physiologic or factual sense to treat peptic ulcers with anything but antibiotics.

The history of our understanding of the cause and appropriate treatment of peptic ulcer has analogues throughout modern science and clinical medicine.[47] What was once taken to be the only truth about a particular condition or treatment is often rejected as false or inaccurate with further experience and upon further reflection. In fact, treatments once thought appropriate and effective are often later proven harmful and contraindicated.

Of course, such is the nature of scientific inquiry and its application in clinical practice. New hypotheses are constantly being tested and new findings incorporated as they are discovered and corroborated. This commitment to inquiry at the core of the scientific method ensures the advancement of knowledge and the development of new approaches, technologies, and understandings. It is the source of scientific and medical progress.

But the acknowledged reality that the process is inherently and unavoidably fraught with uncertainty and mistakes should give us pause when so-called purely factual and indisputable statements are made about the absolute and definitive futility of a therapeutic approach for a given condition. What we understand about various conditions and treatments will always be subject to our continued scrutiny and reevaluation. It is my position that judgments of physiologic futility should be subject to nothing less than the same kind of scrutiny and reevaluation.

Examples of judgments of factual futility ultimately being proved wrong can be found in individual cases as well as at the theoretical level. Instances of misdiagnoses, misprognoses, mistreatments, or general misunderstanding are also well-chronicled in the history of medicine.

The example of Baby K[48] provides an interesting case in point. Oddly, though no one disputed her diagnosis of anencephaly, Baby K lived two and a half years. Despite the fact that anencephaly has been described classically as a condition incompatible with life, we learn through the experience of Baby K that, when treated, at least some anencephalics can live well past their birth.

Hers is a telling example of the tendency to conflate "factual" and normative judgments. Clearly many classic texts that cite anencephaly as a condition incompatible with life mean that it is incompatible with meaningful or worthwhile life, i.e., life worth sustaining by medical means. As it turns out, despite the popular opinion that Baby K's life should not have been sustained, we now know that in point of fact, it was possible to do so. So what was thought to be the case factually has been proved a false assumption primarily influenced by ideas about what normatively ought be the case.

Similar patterns of argumentation and resultant errors can be found in other practice areas as well. A case that stands out in this regard is one in which my colleague Laurie Zoloth-Dorfman consulted.[49] The case involved a 35-year-old-man with AIDS, a request for continued transfusions, an argument about both evaluative and physiologic futility, and a mistake.

James's[50] history included Kaposi's sarcoma, a prior episode of pneumocystis pneumonia (PCP), and a nonresponsive salmonella infection. At the time of the consult, James was pancytopenic and had significant bleeding of unknown etiology. Over the course of 10 days, he had received 200 units of platelets and 50 units of packed red blood cells. The gastroenterologist refused to do an endoscopic procedure because he was afraid it would trigger a fatal bleed. The internist was convinced there was nothing reversible in James's hematological condition, that this was the last event in James's dying process, and that continued blood transfusions would be physiologically futile.

James challenged his internist's conclusion that the transfusions were futile; he consistently felt better after them. In fact, his nurses had come to view the transfusions as comfort measures. In that sense, the case can be understood as a conflict over evaluative futility between James and the nurses on one hand, and the internist on the other. In other words, the question was not whether the transfusions made James feel better, but whether continued transfusions were sufficiently worthwhile or appropriate. James further insisted that to deny him transfusions would be discrimination, and that only he and not the doctors should be allowed to decide how he would die.

The case can also be used to illustrate the extent to which judgments of absolute physiologic futility may turn out to be absolutely wrong. James's gastroenterologist and internist were convinced not only that transfusions were inappropriate, but also that they would not work. They believed with certainty that there was nothing reversible in James's hematological condition. As it turns out, they were wrong, and James lived long enough to prove it. The bioethics committee had recommended that transfusions be continued for a prescribed period of time. A different physician took over the case. In the end, James's bleeding subsided, his condition stabilized, he was able to go home, and he lived for many more months. An eventual endoscopic

procedure revealed that he had not had an irreversible hematological condition, but rather a resolvable bleeding ulcer.

James's case, like countless others that can be cited, reminds us that even
the most well-intentioned judgments of absolute physiologic futility may
turn out to be absolutely wrong. We could not have known prospectively,
but can see clearly retrospectively, that the judgment of physiologic futility was based on incomplete diagnostic information and mistaken clinical
judgment. In this case, and in others, clinical knowledge is necessarily limited, diagnoses and prognoses may be made in error, and judgments of futility may ultimately be proven wrong.

The mere fact that mistakes occur has an impact on our ability to know
with certainty which theories of disease will prove accurate, which interventions will work, and which diagnoses and prognoses will be confirmed.
At issue for our purposes is not the impossible task of preventing mistakes,
but rather the attainable goal of deciding how mistakes, and the related
problem of uncertainty, will be handled. Of critical importance is the recognition that these decisions are rooted in and unavoidably informed by the
particular evaluative and conceptual commitments each of us brings to the
discussion.

Ramifications of Above Criticisms

The range of criticisms detailed in this chapter—from the problems of
objectivity, value neutrality, method, interpretation, and uncertainty, to
mistakes—seriously undercut the popular treatment of physiologic futility
as a sufficient ground for physician unilateral decision making. I contend
that in light of these problems, the practice of privileging or making an exception of physiologic futility and using it to justify physician unilateral decision making ultimately becomes indefensible.

The popular treatment of physiologic futility is misleading because it
misconstrues the process in which the "discovery" of scientific facts is inevitably grounded, by which they are actually constituted, and according to
which they are applied to specific cases. When a physician appeals to the
"scientific or clinical facts" as a justification for unilateral decision making,
she is really appealing to data that have been collected, interpreted, and applied in ways that are subject to critical scrutiny and review, along the lines
suggested in this chapter.

This chapter has shown that the fact/value distinction as traditionally understood, and as adopted in the futility debate, cannot be sustained. In large part the problem is linguistic. When the literature describes judgments of physiologic futility, it typically distinguishes them as factual rather than evaluative. But facts are not so neatly separable from values.

Any "fact" claim can always be broken down into its constitutive parts, that is: data collection plus interpretation plus conclusion plus application. At each juncture in the process, theory-laden and value-laden decisions unavoidably and inevitably have to be made.

The linguistic problem is that "fact" claims are presented as if they refer only to the data underlying them. There is no account of the decisions that are made along the way that ground the fact claim and lead ultimately to the knowledge claim. The futility debate has taken an ill-fated turn by privileging judgments of physiologic futility on the basis of their grounding in scientific fact claims, while at the same time failing to subject those claims to rigorous scrutiny.

When a physician claims that a particular treatment is physiologically futile, she claims, at a chosen level of probability or certainty, that the treatment in question will not produce a relevant physiological effect, that it will be ineffective or will just not work in the circumstances. The predictive claim, by its very nature, cannot be a claim of absolute logical certainty, but only of certainty at a particular confidence level. Consequently, the claim always includes an evaluative component, if only in its choice and interpretation of acceptable certainty and relevance. Accordingly, a physician's selection of a given interpretation can always be challenged on evaluative grounds. A physician's judgment of physiologic futility is also always subject to public challenge on scientific grounds.

In practice, transformations of data into fact claims are regularly and deliberately challenged within the scientific community according to stringent standards of scrutiny and review. Ironically, proposals for physician unilateral decision making on the basis of physiological futility are not even consistent with the framework established by Western science for the careful systematic evaluation of all fact claims. In fact, unilateral decision making threatens to eliminate the possibility of such review.

To exempt physicians from an obligation to publicly and scientifically defend their claims of physiologic futility would be to mistakenly elevate such claims beyond the scope of scientific accountability. In other words, not to subject futility claims to rigorous scientific review forfeits the opportunity to challenge them on the very grounds on which they profess to be reasonable.

This critical analysis of physiologic futility has shown not that facts derived from scientific and clinical data cannot or should not be the basis of treatment decision making, but rather that they cannot and should not be the basis of unilateral physician decision making. Legitimate questions, such as those outlined in this chapter, can be raised about the transformation of data into fact and knowledge claims. Patients, the scientific community, and the broader society should be given an opportunity to raise and pursue these questions.

Patients are entitled to receive an accounting of, and an opportunity to challenge, their physicians's chosen understanding of the data, its appropriate interpretation, its relevance, and its application to the patient's particular circumstance. Physician unilateral decision making on the basis of physiologic futility is unjustified precisely because it would deny patients access to this essential forum. Further, it wrongly presumes that physicians *qua* physicians have exclusive expertise in ascribing meaning, and definitive meaning at that, to data.

At the same time, it would be a mistake to conclude that data collected from scientific trials, in accordance with the scientific method, should have no standing at all. What is left to consider is the appropriate relationship between data derived according to the scientific method, and consensus about its significance both within and among the scientific community, the medical profession, and the lay population.

In Chapter 5, I explore the question of what confirmation on scientific and or consensual grounds would ever be sufficient to warrant denial of patient-requested treatment on the basis of futility. I also consider the clinical and public policy implications of rejecting physician unilateral decision making on the basis of futility. Finally, I suggest an alternative response to conflicts over futility.

❖ 5 ❖

AFTER FUTILITY
A Different Kind of Discourse

THE PREVIOUS FOUR chapters have established that the concept of futility, in either of its common formulations, is an insufficient ground for physician unilateral decision making. That is, physicians would not be justified in refusing unilaterally to offer, provide, or continue treatment based on their opinion that the treatment in question would be futile.

My objection to the popular use and formulation of the concept of futility as outlined in this book has a number of related dimensions. First, I am disturbed by the simplistic terms in which clinicians currently are encouraged to make unilateral treatment decisions: on the grounds of futility. Second, I am skeptical of attempts to divide judgments of futility into factual and evaluative statements. Third, I find untenable the trend towards privileging judgments of so-called factual or physiologic futility. Fourth, I am critical of the process of decision making advocated by the proponents of futility: physician unilateral decision making. I will review briefly each of these critical points in turn and then consider the clinical and public policy implications of my argument.

Reviewing the Problems

First, I am critical of the concept of futility itself. As I have indicated, using the word "futility" without supplying the necessary referent is meaningless and potentially misleading. At the very least, it is necessary to specify the goals with respect to which a treatment is being labelled futile, and to acknowledge whose goals they are. But that is not enough. An examination of the use of the concept of futility in the literature, in the clinical setting, and in the public policy arena evidences an unfortunate practice of stipulating rather than arguing for the goals that should guide medical treatment decisions. Since the selection of goals turns fundamentally on values about which reasonable individuals can and do disagree, this approach remains seriously suspect. What is needed is more focussed public discourse and debate on the values at stake, and collective agreement about how conflicts between values ought be handled.

Another problem with the use of the term "futility" is the way it functions to cloak or obscure other unresolved problems. More specifically, by relying on the cryptic term "futility," much of the discussion deflects attention away from the real and contested questions underlying any conflict over futility and most in need of public debate: what is the place of medicine in society, what is the nature and scope of the authority that society grants to the medical profession, and who among the various stakeholders—physicians, patients, insurers, society—should have the authority to make which kinds of decisions? Rather than debating which particular treatments might be futile under which circumstances, public attention must turn to these critical and prior questions.

Unfortunately, at this point in the debate, asking someone to define futility is tantamount to asking her to define the circumstances under which a physician should have the prerogative to refuse to provide treatment on the basis of futility, even if the treatment is requested expressly by the patient. The word "futility" has achieved such cachet in the clinical environment that it now functions as both a descriptive and a normative signifier. In other words, once a treatment is described as futile, the answer to the normative question of how one ought to respond is implied, if not explicitly proclaimed: If it is futile, physicians need not offer, provide, or continue it. But, contrary to the proposals put forth by futility proponents, this is one of the very questions on which disagreement persists. Again, it is necessary to address directly the prior question of what authority society grants to the medical profession.

My second and third criticisms of the concept of futility are related. I remain skeptical of the almost uniform assumption in the contemporary futility debate that judgments of futility can be categorized according to whether they are factual or evaluative. Further, I find untenable the popular trend towards privileging judgments of so-called factual or physiologic futility. I have concluded that there is not a sufficient philosophically sustainable distinction between factual and evaluative futility that would warrant making an exception of physiologic futility. If physician unilateral decision making on the basis of evaluative futility is unwarranted, then so is physician unilateral decision making on the basis of factual or physiologic futility. I have drawn this conclusion largely by appealing to a social constructionist theory of knowledge and by deconstructing judgments of evaluative and factual futility. At the root of both kinds of futility judgments are significant theoretical and normative value commitments that guide the interpretation of what is futile and what is not.

While the futility literature has for the most part conceded the evaluative component of evaluative futility, it has almost universally failed to recognize the normative import of the unavoidable evaluative component in any scientifically grounded clinical judgment of physiologic or factual futility. As I have demonstrated, even judgments of physiologic or factual futility are fundamentally and unavoidably rooted in value judgments, if only with respect to the appropriate interpretation and application of data and evidence. Conflicts over futility cannot be resolved according to whether the judgments at stake are factual or evaluative. To the contrary, such conflicts signal the need for public dialogue about the real question at stake: whose values should be determinative and on what basis?

My last criticism centers on the proposal of physician unilateral decision making, a mode of decision making sanctioned by many professional position statements and promoted by many of the leading articles in the literature. I have contended that physician unilateral decision making is an excessive and unnecessarily harsh solution to the problem of futility. The practice of physician unilateral decision making damages the trust that is essential to a successful therapeutic relationship between patients and their care providers. Moreover, physician unilateral decision making misconstrues the very grounding of the physician-patient relationship. At its worst, physician unilateral decision making constitutes an unjustified violation of patient autonomy, a return to the oldest form of unjustified paternalism, an unjustified generalization of physician expertise, a breach of the contract between the medical profession and society, and an unwarranted exercise of power. For all of these reasons, given its current definition and use in the futility debate, I have argued that physician unilateral decision making is never justified. At a minimum, patients must always be given an opportunity to participate in the decision making process. But that is not enough.

The opportunity to participate must be genuine and meaningful. Merely disclosing the intent to deny treatment on the grounds of futility, putting patients on notice, or referencing professional position statements or institutional policies is insufficient if physicians ultimately have the power to make and implement treatment decisions on the basis of their judgments of futility. In such an approach concessions to patients constitute only lip service, not actual opportunities to influence, much less control, the decision making process.

The Limited Scope of Criticism

Having reviewed briefly my main areas of concern, I draw attention to a consideration of what I have and have not argued thus far. While I have rejected the simplistic distinction between facts and values that seems so central to the contemporary futility debate, and therefore to the practice of privileging judgments of factual futility, I have not argued that there is no objective medical truth or reality "out there." Instead, I have more modestly claimed that we do not have, and in fact never could have, direct and unmediated access to an objective medical truth or reality.

For some, this will be the hardest part of my argument to accept. After all, many will argue, I cannot possibly mean to suggest that we can know nothing with certainty or that there are no provable scientific facts or truths. I am aware fully of the seductive power of the word "fact" and the degree to which it is an inextricable part of clinical vocabulary, as well as of everyday language. By appealing to a social constructionist theory of knowledge, I am calling not for the rejection of the word, but rather for a more sophisticated and nuanced understanding of the concept, for more public recognition of the unavoidable lenses through which we conceptualize and approach the external world, for more forthright debate about the perspectives we wish to endorse, and for less *de facto* and illegitimate privileging of one perspective at the exclusion of all others.

The social constructionist theory of knowledge, while not perfect, is useful in this regard because it focusses attention on the very issues most in need of our consideration and, significantly, most masked thus far by our debate about the concept of futility. I do not claim that the theory provides all of the answers, but rather that it provides a map of the kinds of questions we need to be asking.

Adopting this theory does not imply that we must abandon all scientific inquiry or lose faith in our ability to know anything with sufficient certainty to act upon it, but that the requisite degree of certainty is something that must be *chosen*; it is not merely *given* by the world "out there." For example, our agreement that under normal circumstances a book will fall to the floor when dropped from the ceiling means simply that we share a high degree of confidence in the ability of our past experience with falling books to predict accurately that the book will fall in this case as well. This reasoning may be applied to the medical context. There may be similar sorts of judgments about which the medical profession and society in general so overwhelmingly agree that they are not only uncontroversial but also perfectly acceptable for the medical profession to act upon. But the warrant for acting on such judgments comes not from some intrinsic quality of the judgment itself, but rather from our agreement to sanction it. What is problematic in the futility debate is the undefended privileging of the medical profession's perspective without the necessary next step, that is, investigation of the degree to which society shares, respects, or endorses that perspective.

It is important to note that I have intentionally and carefully not argued against a physician's right ever to refuse to offer, provide, or continue treatments desired by patients. Nor have I argued against society's role in setting limits to what treatments patients can expect reasonably to receive. Rather, I have objected only to physician unilateral decision making on the basis of futility.

Thus far I have argued that when there is a conflict between a patient and a physician over either evaluative or physiologic futility, physician unilateral decision making on the grounds of the contested judgment of futility is unjustified. In either instance, the patient is entitled, at the very least, to be included as a genuine participant in the decision making process. Moreover, the patient is entitled to challenge the basis for the physician's claim that the treatment is futile.

I have established that the patient is better qualified than the physician to determine the meaning and value a particular intervention will have in the patient's life, i.e., whether it is evaluatively futile. And the patient is entitled to an opportunity to challenge the physician's determination that a particular intervention will work or be effective, i.e., whether it is physiologically futile, even though the physician inevitably has more clinical experience than the patient. The physician's claim to privileged judgment is always subject to challenge. To the extent that the physician's judgment of physiologic futility is reducible to an evaluative judgment not endorsed by the patient, the patient is entitled to reclaim the prerogative to make her own evaluative judgments. And, to the extent that the physician's judgment relies on the collection, interpretation, and application of data, the patient is entitled to challenge, within the stipulated scientific framework, the value judgments that guide the physician's judgment at each of those stages.

I do not suggest that if the patient successfully challenges or rejects the physician's futility judgment, the patient is then necessarily entitled to receive the treatment from the physician, but merely that the physician cannot unilaterally refuse to provide the treatment on futility grounds.

Alternative Grounds for Refusal: The Role of Public Discourse, Social Consensus, and Public Policy

Having rejected the use of the concept of futility to justify physician unilateral decision making, I will now investigate the source of other, viable justifications for refusing treatments desired by patients. Rejecting physician unilateral decision making on the grounds of futility does not entail that physicians must always comply with every patient request for treatment, nor does it reduce physicians to mere technicians subject to the whims of the lay population. Rather, it enables physicians to act as professionals with clinical and moral integrity—but only within the reasonable limits set in partnership with the lay population and grounded in the stipulated frame of Western science. Of course, the phrase "reasonable limits" might seem initially to beg the question of what the limits might be. But my phrasing is intentional, since the reasonable limits cannot be known *a priori*, but rather must be derived organically from collective dialogue.

The Social Contract and the Role of Social Discourse

It has become commonplace to argue that medicine is an inherently moral enterprise. What has been missing in the futility debate is the recognition that medicine is also essentially, and unavoidably, a social practice. The practice of medicine exists within a particular social context, is informed inevitably and appropriately by the values of that context, and is constrained ultimately by the parameters set by that context.

That is why the question of whether physicians should be empowered to make unilateral decisions on the basis of futility cannot be answered exclusively by the medical profession. Any question about the limits that should be set to the scope and practice of medicine must ultimately be answered not just by medicine but by society as well. Such a question must be asked and debated publicly, in the context of a critical and prior discussion about the nature of the relationship between the medical profession and society.

One of the most promising ways to understand the relationship between the medical profession and society comes from the idea of a partnership or social contract. The idea of a social contract that defines and governs the relation between the professions and society has many sources. I draw here specifically on the approach employed by Robert M. Veatch.[1] Veatch argues that a viable medical ethics cannot be based exclusively on professionally generated standards and codes. Instead, it must be grounded in something more fundamental, something beyond itself. The social contract or covenant between the medical profession and society properly establishes the nature and scope of the medical enterprise, the role-specific duties of physicians, and the standards of acceptable behavior to which physicians will be held accountable. The social contract establishes, in essence, the framework within which the profession is given license to practice and the source and justification for the rules governing such practice.

I find the social contract approach to be one of the most viable ways to locate the source of authority and justification for medical practice. This approach needs further exploration and development. But, I submit, vigorous, public debate over the specific meaning and terms of the contract between the medical profession and society would be far more productive and to the point than the debate over the merits of medical futility judgments. We could thus more fruitfully return to such underlying questions as: What is the nature and extent of authority granted to physicians by society? What conditions, if any, are societally imposed on the practice of medicine? What practices are physicians socially sanctioned to engage in? What obligations do physicians have to society? What reasonable expectations should physicians have of society and patients? What should be expected of physicians? What mechanism best stimulates dialogue and addresses points of conflict between the medical profession and society?

The idea of the social contract has already been applied to the futility debate. Veatch and Mason Spicer, for example, argue that physicians incur particular role-specific obligations in exchange for the monopoly society has granted them over knowledge about, access to, and skill in the use of life saving medical technology.[2] That is, in exchange for the control they have been granted over diagnostic procedures, therapeutic treatments, pharmaceutical agents, et cetera, and in exchange for their license to practice, physicians owe patients and society something—namely, provision of those medical goods and services to patients in need under certain agreed upon circumstances.[3]

Key to this approach is recognition that the particulars and circumstances must be established as part of the social contract between society and the medical profession, rather than by members of the medical profession alone.

In this context the principle of fidelity—i.e., the commitment to promise-keeping—emerges as a far more viable ground than patient autonomy for obligating physicians to provide requested treatments they might otherwise deem futile. As already discussed, the principle of respect for autonomy by itself can only ground a right of noninterference as opposed to a positive right of entitlement. As such, the principle of respect for autonomy can only take us so far in the futility debate. Respect for autonomy drives my argument against the unwanted imposition of a physician's value judgment on a patient. And the principle of fidelity picks up where autonomy leaves off, charting a potential path for patients to access services that physicians may have an obligation to provide despite their own individual evaluative judgments. Of course, specifying the precise circumstances under which a physician might be so obligated is a difficult task. But it begins with a certain kind of dialogue, a certain kind of discourse.

Social discourse is one of the most important mechanisms for clarifying and modifying the terms of the contract and identifying the nature and scope of promises made. And it is meaningful social discourse that is most significantly lacking in the futility debate. The problem with the concept of futility is not that it is used to limit the treatment that patients can expect to receive, but rather that it limits treatment on questionable, even professionally idiosyncratic grounds, without meaningful public involvement or endorsement.

What has been missing is prior public discourse and decision making about the grounds on which we could collectively and prospectively authorize physicians to refuse to provide treatment desired by patients. Inclusive public democratic discourse aimed at identifying our collective concerns, values, and priorities, and at establishing the points on which we do and do not have consensus will move the debate forward on more defensible grounds. When there is agreement among the scientific community, the medical profession, and the lay population, physicians can set limits to medical treatment without conflict and without violating their promises. Only when there is disagreement does the conflict at issue in the futility debate arise. And, not coincidentally, it is at this level that physician unilateral decision making has been proposed. But the conflict cannot be resolved by fiat. A different kind of discourse and process will be necessary for physicians to have the authority to refuse.

In what follows I briefly consider three possible grounds for physician refusal to provide requested treatment that might emerge from such public discourse: respect for physician autonomy and integrity, relevance as an example of overwhelming consensus, and concerns for social justice. Then, I outline an alternative response to physician unilateral decision making that I recommend should be employed in the absence of public consensus about grounds on which physicians may refuse to provide treatment.

Public Policy on the Basis of Respect for Physician Autonomy and Integrity: Professional Codes and Standards

One of the defining characteristics of a profession is its ability to develop its own code of ethics and standards for acceptable practice. This explains in part the emergence of futility position statements by medical specialty groups. But according to the social contract model, codes and standards developed by the medical profession, like those developed by any other profession, must not only meet with professional approval, but must also be consistent with the mandate given to the profession by society.

Increasingly, even the strongest proponents of futility have begun to recognize the need for public involvement and social consensus in this regard. But, I would argue, the role and standing of society has yet to be adequately understood or addressed.

For example, while noting the need for society's ultimate endorsement, Schneiderman and Jecker maintain that it is the responsibility of the medical profession to proactively take the initiative, define the parameters, and set the standards with regard to the problem of medical futility. Theirs is not a model of genuine collaborative exchange, but rather one in which the presumed experts set the terms that they hope society will come to endorse under their responsible tutelage. A review of the steps they propose for resolution of the futility debate makes their vision of public dialogue perfectly clear. As discussed earlier, they begin by stipulating their own proposed definition of medical futility: that which fails to achieve the goals of medicine. Next, they call for an effort to secure physician agreement as to what counts as a minimum probability or minimal quality of benefit. They then call for the resultant definition to be introduced into practice. Only after all of the most important work has been done, they recommend seeking to educate and obtain the concurrence of society at large by declaring these standards of care openly, as institutional policies for the information of the public (including legislatures and governmental agencies) and as guidelines for the courts.[4]

One might question the intention and reasoning behind such an approach. Why should the medical profession take responsibility for resolving the problem of medical futility in this way? In light of this question the following admission by Schneiderman and Jecker becomes most interesting.

> We acknowledge that there is no present consensus within the medical profession about the exact dimensions of futility. . . . Can the medical community achieve a consensus and put forward for public assessment a definition of medical futility? One answer is to point out that the courts will not await such a development, but rather they will continue to make ad hoc emotionally propelled decisions, or . . . decisions based on idiosyncratic interpretations of federal statutues . . . causing physicians and patients to become mired in ever more intractable confusion. Therefore, in our view, the responsibility rests with the medical profession to take the initiative by offering specific standards and guidelines in the hope of first achieving consensus within the medical community and ultimately gaining acceptance in society at large.[5]

I would suggest that this is a rather impoverished view of the necessary role society and broad social discourse have in resolving an issue of such contentiousness. It is a proposed path to resolution that reveals more about the stark power differentials and strong interests at stake than about a commitment to take seriously the claims of competing points of view. This failing is particularly unfortunate in light of the acknowledged reality that there is no consensus on core issues in the futility debate either within the profession or between the profession and society. A far more defensible approach would recognize that the only legitimate standards are based not only on professional conceptions of the worthy ends of medicine, but on socially generated and validated conceptions as well.[6]

At issue, of course, is how to engage the profession and the lay public in meaningful discourse. This issue merits much more deliberate consideration. Preliminary guidance can be found in the works of Jonathon D. Moreno[7] and Daniel Yankelovich,[8] who each contemplates the process and meaning of the development of social consensus; in the Oregon Prioritization Process,[9] which employed focus groups to contemplate the values that should undergird any policy of health care rationing; and in the grassroots bioethics movement,[10] which has been successful in stimulating discussion in the community about ethical issues.

One thing is clear: the scope of public discourse must be sufficiently broad to encompass a review of the range of justifications offered for positions taken. In specifying the kinds of assessments that should be open to public scrutiny, Howard Brody offers a helpful beginning. He distinguishes between power that is shared appropriately with patients and power that is rightly owned by physicians. Like Schneiderman and Jecker, Brody thinks that physicians should have the unilateral power to make judgments of futility and withhold an intervention "when it can reasonably be predicted to produce no acceptable therapeutic outcome."[11] But Brody makes clear that the profession's determinations may not meet with public endorsement. For that reason he insists,

> Whenever possible, such decisions should be based on value judgments and empirical data that can be presented for public discussion and challenge.[12]

For Brody, as a condition of owned power, the public has a right to review and criticize both the evaluative and empirical judgments made by the medical profession.

> The . . . disclosure required by owned power is for the medical profession to establish an open process for defending judgments of futility for certain classes of patients and interventions. . . . The value assumptions as well as the empirical observations must be candidly reported if the goal of owned power and full public dialogue is to be met.[13]

Clearly in dispute in the futility debate and most in need of public discussion is a consideration of the standards of care that will be socially sanctioned and the source and basis for the standards that will be accepted. In general, society has taken seriously the importance of protecting the integrity of the medical profession[14] and respecting the integrity and autonomy of individual physicians. For example, it has long been established that an individual patient cannot compel an individual physician to perform an abortion if the physician is morally opposed to abortion. On the other hand, the range of explanations a physician can offer justifiably for refusal on such moral grounds is fairly narrow. We generally accept that a physician competent to treat AIDS patients cannot refuse to treat an AIDS patient on the basis of his personal feelings and fears about the disease, and that a physician cannot refuse to treat a patient on the basis of the patient's race, class, gender, or sexual orientation. Such refusals would be considered discriminatory and could be challenged legally.

Application of the discussion of physician autonomy and integrity to the futility debate has yet to be explored adequately.[15] Obviously, physician refusal to provide treatment on the basis of physician autonomy, integrity, and moral belief is conceptually distinct from physician refusal on the basis of futility. Refusal on these alternative grounds may well be defensible. Ultimately, however, to be acceptable, such grounds would be subject to social review and approval. They could not be asserted and imposed solely by the medical profession.

As a society we would surely want to find some mechanism for taking into account the deeply held moral beliefs of physicians. After all, both patients and physicians should have the prerogative to make their own evaluative judgments and to act accordingly. The question is whether physicians should be empowered to impose their own evaluative judgments on their patients, and what would constitute doing so.

It is accepted widely that while physicians may act in accordance with their own deeply held moral beliefs, they also have a duty individually and collectively not to abandon patients. So, if a physician has a personal moral objection to the treatment a patient insists upon, transfer of care to another willing and competent physician is regarded as an acceptable option. In fact, the availability of transfer is viewed traditionally as a necessary condition of a physician's termination of a patient relationship. Importantly, we accept this option out of our respect for the individual physician's autonomy, not out of our acceptance of futility judgments as a permissible ground for ending the physician-patient relationship.

The issue becomes much less clear, however, when care cannot be transferred because no other physician is willing or able to accept the case. In those much more difficult cases, the role-specific duties of the individual physician and the medical profession at large are more directly called into question. The question of how to frame such role-specific duties—especially when the choice is between violating a patient's most fundamental beliefs and desires, and violating a physician's sense of professional and personal integrity—requires attention and can only legitimately be resolved at the level of social policy. To be justifiable, any parameters defined or exceptions made to a physician's role-specific duty must be subject to public review and approval. This is one essential reason why futility conflicts cannot be resolved exclusively and unilaterally by individual physicians or even by the medical profession alone.

Public Policy on the Basis of Consensus:
The Example of Relevance

Public policy recognizes another legitimate instance of physician refusal to provide treatment desired by patients: when there is overwhelming consensus supporting the refusal. Such consensus evolves in different ways, takes different forms, and exists to various degrees. One example of a category on which we have overwhelming consensus is the concept of relevance. If there is overwhelming consensus in both the medical profession and the broader lay population about the absence of any causal relationship between a given treatment and the goal for which it is being considered, we agree without hesitation, much less serious consideration, that the patient cannot compel a physician to provide it. In such cases, physicians are sanctioned simply to refuse to provide the requested treatment. Of course, patients could always later challenge whether a physician's claim accurately reflected an overwhelming consensus. But we presume that if the physician's refusal genuinely reflected an overwhelming consensus of the medical profession and the lay population, it would ultimately, albeit retrospectively, be formally endorsed.

Accordingly, we agree that a physician would not be obligated to amputate a patient's arm to relieve a headache because there is no plausible relevance between the treatment, amputation, and the goal, relief of headache. The physician could refuse to provide the requested treatment, and explain his justification. In this paradigmatic case, social consensus confirms and therefore endorses the medical profession's evaluative judgment of appropriate limits. A specific written policy permitting physicians to refuse to amputate limbs to relieve headaches would not be required, nor would mandatory prospective review by an outside body.

Such strong social determination of a treatment's irrelevance may at first appear to be a fact known with a high degree of certainty. But as I use the term, relevance simply means that the evaluative component of the knowledge claim in question is supported by such overwhelming and widespread consensus, that it is rendered practically invisible. This leaves the impression that the claim is based exclusively on indisputable data. In fact, the refusal is justified not because the treatment actually "is" absolutely irrelevant, but rather because we overwhelming agree that it is so. Our overwhelming agreement serves as endorsement of the physician's refusal.

The difference between claiming that a particular treatment is physiologically futile and claiming that it is irrelevant is nothing more than a difference in the degree of public consensus and endorsement. Irrelevance takes several steps beyond an individual physician's judgment of physiologic futility by insisting that the evaluative component of the judgment be supported by the broadest possible consensus. It is not enough that the individual physician deems the treatment to be inappropriate, or that his peers concur. Rather, the physician must argue either that there already is overwhelming consensus about the treatment's inappropriateness both in the medical profession and in the lay population, or that the case is so obvious that such consensus would inevitably follow a public discussion of the matter.

In the absence of actual or expected consensus, the validity and therefore the normative weight of a single individual physician's knowledge claim diminishes substantially. Only on the basis of overwhelming consensus can a physician ever have sufficient ground to refuse, without reproach, to provide a treatment desired by a patient.

If there is controversy regarding the appropriateness of a particular treatment for a given condition, or if the physician is merely articulating his own beliefs or defending a particular side in the debate, he cannot claim that there is or would inevitably be overwhelming consensus on the matter, and that his refusal is therefore socially sanctioned. Admittedly, well-meaning physicians might be tempted to abuse the concept of consensus by insisting that it exists where it clearly does not in order to bolster support for their refusal. The best safeguard against this is a reliable system of review and oversight in which claims about the existence of consensus could always be challenged.

As I have used it, relevance describes one extreme end of a spectrum of consensus by which physician refusal could be supported and socially sanctioned. Consensus is so overwhelming at that end that the authority of claims backed by such widespread agreement seems obvious and indisputable. At the other extreme end are issues that have not yet been anticipated, adequately addressed, or clearly resolved—i.e., issues on which consensus is lacking. Somewhere in the middle of the spectrum of consensus are issues that we have explicitly addressed and to which we have formulated specific responses.

The increasingly popular professional standards and practice guidelines are an example of this midpoint on the consensus spectrum. Such standards and guidelines, if they have been subject to genuine and meaningful public review and thus represent an evolving consensus, can also support a justification of physician refusal. In applicable cases, a physician would be socially sanctioned to refuse to provide a requested treatment not because he or his peers deemed refusal to be appropriate, but rather because we agreed prospectively to support his refusal in such instances. He can point to our endorsement of the standards and guidelines as evidence.

This discussion of the role of consensus in establishing a socially sanctioned basis for physician refusal illustrates the most serious problem with physician unilateral decision making on the basis of futility. Such consensus is plainly lacking. Further, it must be stressed that, even if such consensus could eventually be established, unilateral decision making would still remain unacceptable. Disclosure to the patient and documentation of the reasons for refusal—treatment irrelevance—are always necessary.

Public Policy on the Basis of Social Justice Concerns

The concept of relevance as determined by overwhelming consensus clarifies and limits the options available to physicians and society when patients make demands for treatment. Once treatment relevance is established, a conflict between a physician and patient becomes an evaluative conflict over futility, and the physician has no authority to refuse exclusively on the grounds of futility. Likewise, once the relevance of a treatment is established, there are only limited grounds on which society may justifiably intervene to override a patient's evaluative assessment of a treatment's worth.

With respect to overriding a patient's assessment of a treatment's worth, society has standing only on social justice grounds. In other words, society never has authority to determine a treatment's intrinsic worth for any given patient; the prerogative to make such an evaluative judgment is reserved for that patient herself. On the other hand, if social consensus deems certain treatments to be insufficiently worth pursuing *with respect to other competing social goods*, rather than insufficiently worth it *per se*, a limit can justifiably be set to treatments individual patients can reasonably expect to receive. Only society, not the individual physician, or even the medical profession at large, can legitimately set limits on evaluative grounds to what individuals can expect to receive as parties to the social contract.

The final viable alternative ground for setting limits to the provision of treatment requested by patients is our developed and shared conception of the requirements of social justice. Only from this perspective can the larger community legitimately impose limits on what the individual can expect to receive from the collective.

I contend that appeals to social justice rather than to futility provide the most promising and defensible strategy for setting reasonable limits in medicine. Furthermore, I maintain that the best solution to the futility problem in the clinic and at the bedside is to resolve the justice problem at the societal level. Systematically and prospectively setting limits to the interventions that will be offered under particular circumstances is far more justifiable than having individual physicians arbitrarily and inconsistently apply inevitably value-loaded futility judgments in the clinic or at the bedside.

The kind of public discourse I am calling for extends far beyond that which has started to occur at the individual institutional and community level.[16] I envision a process of public discourse along the lines of that used in the Oregon health care prioritization project.[17] Oregon's use of focus groups—composed of professionals and members of the lay population, and charged with considering not only what health care services they valued most, but also what values they thought should undergird the provision of health care services in their state—offers a promising model. Similar public discussion of the essential questions of social justice would more directly respond to the concerns that really fuel the futility debate: How should the needs and desires of the individual be weighed against the needs and desires of the community? What would be a fair and equitable distribution of our collective resources, both human and financial?

Setting limits based on consensually agreed upon answers to these questions would be far more honest and defensible than physician unilateral decision making based on futility. It would be far more honest and defensible to say to the family of a patient in a persistent vegetative state that we have collectively and prospectively decided not to fund dialysis for PVS patients, than to say to the family that dialysis for their loved one would be futile. Denying dialysis on the grounds of social justice rather than futility would clarify the issues really at stake, and would introduce a level of accountability that extends far beyond a single physician's judgment.

In some sense, the very existence of the contemporary futility debate can be understood as symptomatic of our failure to engage in public discourse regarding how limits can and should be set in the health care arena. If the necessary discourse had already taken place and a societal consensus had already been forged regarding limits, the futility debate might never have arisen, and undoubtedly would not have taken its current form. Precisely because we have steadfastly avoided necessary public limit setting, physicians have been left with the responsibility of making *de facto* policy decisions at the bedside.

The relationship between individual physician decision making at the bedside and collective deliberation and resolution at the policy level is sorely in need of correction. Individual physicians, or even hospitals, should not be asked to make decisions in a vacuum. We have a communal responsibility to tackle these difficult questions before they arise in the individual physician-patient encounter. Public discourse should establish the framework within which individual medical decisions are made. In other words, consensually agreed upon *a priori* limits may appropriately be set, on the grounds of justice, to constrain the options available to both the physician and the patient.

Responding to Value Claims Not Represented in Social Consensus

A question that will arise inevitably in the context of inclusive public discourse and prospective decision making is what protection, if any, ought to exist to protect the minority whose perspective is not reflected by social consensus. Public debate and policy making must incorporate the decision of how to respond to patients who insist upon treatment deemed by social consensus to be insufficiently worth pursuing with respect to other competing social goods.

What if, for example, some families insist that their loved ones would view life in a persistent vegetative state as intrinsically worth preserving? Should the patients' wishes and beliefs be overridden because they are not in accordance with the societal consensus? Should their wishes carry any more weight if they are religiously motivated? Should their wishes be honored only if patients are able to pay for the desired services? These questions are the most difficult to answer in the futility debate and the most in need of further public reflection.

Several interesting responses to the dilemma of balancing an interest in broad social consensus with an interest in respecting the dissenting minority perspective might offer guidance in the futility debate. The New Jersey Declaration of Death Act[18] stands as a notable example that takes seriously the notion that the minority perspective must be honored, so much so that it includes a religious exemption to protect those whose beliefs would be violated by the imposition of a brain death standard of death. The New Jersey statute explicitly recognizes that the determination of death is not solely a medical judgment about a biological fact, but rather a value judgment informed by one's fundamental beliefs.[19]

The parallels to the futility debate are striking. At the heart of both the brain death debate and the futility debate are questions of expertise and power: Who should be empowered to make judgments and decisions? Are they at root medical or moral judgments and decisions? What sort of expertise do such decisions require? Whose perspective should trump?

In light of the New Jersey religious exemption, it might be argued that a similar exemption should protect minority perspectives not represented by societal consensus reached in a justice-based approach to limit setting. So, for example, even if there were broad societal consensus on the grounds of justice that communal funds not be used to support dialysis for PVS patients (a currently debated issue), it might be argued that an exemption should be crafted to allow the family with a minority perspective potential recourse. Perhaps access would be permitted if the family paid the costs and if the capacity existed to provide dialysis without jeopardizing others.

But such a solution is not without problems. First, how do we define a "minority" perspective? Do all dissenting positions qualify? Second, what grounds would be sufficient to compel a physician to provide the treatment rejected by the majority but desired by the minority? Third, would a patient's ability to pay be a necessary condition for compelling a physician to provide the desired treatment? These important questions about physicians' role-specific duties must be addressed and resolved in public discourse.

Alternatively, one might propose grounding the minority's right of access in the social contract between society and the medical profession and in the promises made by the latter as a condition of the contract. One might argue that because patients with minority perspectives have no other means of access to the treatment they view as necessary (either morally or medically), physicians must either make the treatment available themselves, or find another physician who is willing to take over care of the patient. Veatch and Mason Spicer[20] argue that, in certain limited circumstances, when the choice comes down to violating a physician's conscience or ending the life of a patient who, contrary to the physician, holds a minority belief in the intrinsic value and meaning of even mere biological existence, the decision should be made to err on the side of life.

They use a Rawlsian veil of ignorance to defend their position, suggesting that if we were ignorant of our own specific situation, and therefore didn't know whether we agreed with the majority or minority, we would choose a system of licensing physicians that included a mechanism for protecting the interests of the minority. So, in part, because we would want the treatment made available to us if we were the ones with the unusual desire, we are inclined to ensure that it be available to those with minority views.

Importantly, the impetus and justification for creating such a mechanism would be not patient autonomy, but rather the importance of fidelity, i.e., promise-keeping according to the terms of the contract with society. Physicians would be obligated to provide treatment in such cases not simply because patients with minority beliefs desired them, but rather because by accepting a license that gave them monopoly control, they made certain commitments or promises.

Veatch and Mason Spicer go on to argue that most rational individuals would want the medical profession to make certain publicly funded interventions available in limited circumstances, even if the medical profession judged the desirability of the interventions differently. They maintain that if there were an equitable funding source, physicians would have an obligation to provide the care as a condition of their contract with society. So, for example, if Helga Wanglie had purchased a PVS insurance rider to cover the cost of care for her in a persistent vegetative state, she should be entitled to receive that treatment from her physicians, even if they themselves would recommend against it.

But what about desired interventions that are not equitably funded? Should minority views only be respected if there is equitable funding for the treatments they desire? Should ability to pay really determine the degree to which wishes, particularly minority wishes, will be honored? Should funding really be the final determinant of physician obligation? Again, these difficult questions must be addressed and resolved at the public policy level.

One possible solution would be to designate a certain percentage of public funds to cover the expense of respecting minority perspectives. Or perhaps, as Veatch has suggested, we could allocate to each citizen an annual fixed dollar amount for purchasing a basic package of health care according to their own values and priorities.[21] So, the Helga Wanglies of the world might choose a package that included ventilatory support for PVS patients but excluded other services that were less valuable to them.

Similarly, we might encourage minority groups to develop their own health insurance plans in order to fund the kind of medical treatment they deem appropriate. As Stephen G. Post argues,

> [T]hose with expensive beliefs should take responsibility for them, forming their separate managed care organizations. . . . [I]n a just health care system, believers who reject the wider society's accepted standards of medical futility, definitions of death, and blood use have no claim on nonbelievers for a financial blank check. The individual or sect holding an expensive belief must pay for it. Otherwise, the wider society is held hostage to any and all creeds.[22]

Post cites the Ohio Amish community who have their own insurance pool and who collectively make decisions about how their shared resources will be spent. This is a promising public policy proposal that merits further social reflection.

A final question worth raising in public discourse and debate regards the nature of the minority perspective typically manifested in conflicts over futility. Though there are no known empirical studies documenting this phenomenon, it would be interesting to reflect on the extent to which spiritually or religiously motivated requests for treatment play a role in futility conflicts in this country. Not coincidentally, patients guided by a strong spiritual belief in the ability of God to heal, in the meaning that can be found in suffering, or in the preciousness and sanctity of even biologic life itself, seem to be disproportionately represented in the group of patients who demand treatment that the physician may deem futile, or that society may deem insufficiently worth the expenditure of our collective resources.

Considering the degree to which patients' spiritual beliefs guide their perception of the meaning of life, death, pain, suffering, healing, et cetera, we might consider at the public policy level what different weight, if any, we want to accord to spiritual beliefs. Should we, could we, defensibly privilege the spiritually or religiously motivated request for continued treatment? Does the basis of the request matter? Or should all requests for treatment be treated the same? Again, these questions merit more deliberate social reflection and debate.

I have thus far considered three possible alternatives to futility as grounds for physician refusal that are worth considering in public discourse and debate. In the absence of viable grounds for physician refusal that are derived from social discourse and encoded in public policy, there is an important alternative that must be explored.

Another Alternative: Genuine Conversation

Sometimes it will be necessary for physicians to act in the absence of clear social consensus and public policy. It may take time to resolve thoughtfully and equitably the challenging issues discussed above. Further, there will always be areas in which consensus has not developed, if only because advances in technology or the emergence of new diseases always raise new questions and dilemmas. The ever changing terrain of health care decision making can by illustrated by two notable recent examples: the development of the technological means to sustain life in a persistent vegetative state and the advent of the AIDS epidemic. In each case, new questions arose and consensus at the public policy level was slow to evolve. So even if we have inclusive public discourse, and establish prospectively the grounds of physician integrity, treatment irrelevance, and social justice according to which limits could justifiably be set, we will not be able to anticipate every dilemma that may arise in the clinic and at the bedside. For such circumstances, in the absence of clear consensus and guidance, I propose the following alternative to physician unilateral decision making on the grounds of futility.

It is necessary to consider what responses I have left available to physicians once the possibility of unilateral decision making on the basis of futility is excluded. In light of my critical analysis, in the absence of other consensually agreed upon grounds for refusal, how ought a physician respond to patient demands for treatment the physician deems futile?

I contend that a commitment to a particular kind of conversation in the clinic, at the bedside, and at the policy level would offer a far more defensible response than unilateral decision making on the basis of futility. Given the lack of public consensus regarding the definition of futility, the selection of goals of treatment, or the criteria by which supposed futility could be judged, the normative call for careful deliberate conversation seems obvious, though it has not received nearly as much attention as unilateral decision making.

I have already argued that as an answer to the question of what a physician should do when faced with unrealistic, yet unrelenting patient expectations and demands, physician unilateral decision making is an excessively and unnecessarily harsh response. A far more effective approach in nearly every case is to engage in honest, meaningful conversation—not a monologue—using what I will call dialogue, moral suasion, and transparent disclosure. Let me break down the components of this recommendation.

Dialogue

By insisting upon genuine dialogue instead of silence, secrecy, or one-sided disclosures, I am positing what I take to be a healthier and more defensible model of physician-patient interaction. One can draw on a range of ethical arguments in support of this model. Not only would the interaction be more likely to succeed, but each party would be more trusting of the other, and would likely feel that the other was more properly motivated and cognizant of particular role-specific duties that marked the boundaries of the relationship.

As already discussed, after recognizing the potential dangers of the extreme form of unilateral decision making, some futility proponents have seen the need for modifications and have recommended against silence and secrecy in favor of frank discussion.[23] But the modifications often remain insufficient. As this honest quotation from Howard Brody makes clear, the modifications are intentionally limited in their aim.

> The physician must inform the patient or family when an intervention is being withheld on the basis of futility. This is different from seeking consent; *it is simply a courteous disclosure of relevant information.* The physician accepts full responsibility for the decision and in no way seeks to involve the patient or family in the decision-making process, but nevertheless he makes clear that the decision is being made without any attempt at concealment or misrepresentation.[24]

The meaning and intent of such "courteous disclosure" support a model of unilateral, not bilateral decision making under which the physician quite deliberately retains the ultimate decision making prerogative.

I suggest genuine conversation with a different intention and goal. The kind of dialogue I have in mind would not merely convey information regarding the physician's assessment and intended plan of action. Merely informing a patient that a particular treatment is futile in the physician's opinion does nothing to advance the discussion or resolve the ethical dilemma.

Rather, conversation enables the physician and the patient to convey information, to fill gaps in each other's knowledge, to share their potentially divergent perspectives, to review their expectations, to challenge their assumptions, and, subsequently, to explore together what the best course of action might be.

For such a conversation to be useful, it must be structured as a genuine dialogue. As such, it must involve a real sharing of perspective and position, a willingness on the part of patient and physician to subject their claims to examination and review. To be meaningful, it must openly and deliberately address the possible goal(s) in light of which the treatment in question might or might not be futile.

Moral Suasion

In the context of this kind of discourse and partnership, moral suasion can be both indicated and appropriate. Physicians have a role-specific duty to consider their patients' best interests above all else. Based on this duty, on their presumed possession of far more clinical experience and expertise than the average member of the lay population, and on their more direct access to relevant data, physicians can attempt appropriately to persuade patients that a particular treatment is in their best interest. In fact, most patients rely on their physicians for clear, well-reasoned recommendations based on their greater experience and expertise. But making a recommendation and using moral suasion to encourage patient acceptance is far different from unilaterally imposing a decision upon a resisting or unwitting patient.

My call for genuine conversation runs exactly counter to the popular proposal of physician unilateral decision making on the grounds of futility. In fact, labelling as futile a particular treatment course for a given patient or patient population tends to stop, rather than start, conversations. The implied message is that there is nothing else for a physician to say to a patient. Judging a treatment to be futile is presumed to justify foregoing not only the treatment itself, but the conversation about it as well.

This is perhaps one of the most damaging consequences of the popular proposal for unilateral decision making based on futility. Futility tends to turn physicians away from exploratory conversation at the precise moment when it is most needed. Under my proposed solution, when a physician finds herself thinking about a given treatment's futility, she will recognize the occasion for initiating a special kind of conversation with her patient, and she will understand that it is her responsibility to do so.

Transparent Disclosure

To describe the physician-patient dialogue I have in mind, I borrow a concept from Howard Brody's earlier work on informed consent.[25] In response to the question of what constitutes adequate disclosure in the process of informed consent, Brody proposed a "transparency model": a physician can know he has met the standard of adequate disclosure if he has successfully made his clinical reasoning transparent to the patient.[26] This means that he has successfully conveyed the basis of his diagnosis and prognosis, including the reasons for his choice of data, his interpretation of the data, and his beliefs about the data's relevance and applicability.

Employment of this model would contribute much toward resolving seemingly intractable conflicts of futility in the clinical setting. If physicians made their reasoning transparently clear to patients and if patients had the opportunity to do the same, dialogue would be far more productive, and intractable conflicts far less frequent.

By engaging in such dialogue, rather than hiding in silence, or talking at or past one another, physicians and patients would tackle the source of potential conflict head-on. That is, rather than merely stating a preferred course of action, each would make clear and accessible their reasons for selecting their preferred goals.

Transparent disclosure could enable patients and physicians to answer a variety of questions. What metaphysical, epistemological, and normative commitments guide their reasoning? What is the meaning of the illness or the suffering? What kinds of lives do they consider worth living? What background beliefs do they hold? What past experiences shape their perspective? What meaning do they ascribe to the intervention in question and why? What non-medical considerations inform their perspective? Which risks do they judge worth or not worth taking, and why? What p values have they implicitly selected, that is, what level of confidence do they seek, and why? What scientific and clinical data are considered relevant, and why? Is there consensus about the appropriate interpretation and application of the data?

I contend that if physicians and patients refocus the dialogue on goals, and make their reasoning process not only more apparent, but transparent, they will seldom find themselves in intractable conflicts over futility. I submit that more often than not, either the physician and patient will reach an understanding or compromise that ameliorates the conflict, or, much more rarely, one of the parties will decide to leave the relationship. With intractable conflicts over futility the exception and not the rule, both the need and the justification for physician unilateral decision making diminishes substantially.

In fact, in most circumstances, the kind of dialogue I recommend will be the most productive solution to the problem. Interestingly, though not surprisingly, two popularly cited studies of patient decision making after full disclosure of diagnosis and extremely poor prognosis revealed that 88% and 96% of patients, respectively, elected to forego rather than to receive aggressive life sustaining measures.[27] Persistent demands for aggressive treatment were simply not the norm. A more recent study further suggests that the actual frequency with which patients persistently demand treatment deemed futile by physicians may in fact be low.[28]

While intractable futility conflicts have captured the imagination and interest of clinicians and ethicists alike, most cases are in fact resolved when treated with careful attention and conversation. And they are resolved more often than not with a decision to forego rather than continue further medical interventions.

Resolving Any Remaining Intractable Futility Conflicts

I have reviewed three alternatives to grounding physician unilateral refusal to provide treatment on the basis of futility. I expect these to emerge out of the process of public discourse and debate. I have also outlined an alternative to physician unilateral decision making on the basis of futility in the absence of public consensus and public policy. I now offer a preliminary sketch of the mechanisms I propose for the resolution of any remaining intractable conflicts over futility.

No Grounds for Physician Unilateral Decision Making

By now it should be clear that given the current usage of the term "unilateral," I find physician unilateral decision making on any grounds to be unacceptable. At the very least, patients must always be given an opportunity to participate meaningfully in the decision making process. Further, as a condition of the social contract, physicians are accountable to the broader society for the decisions they make. Since there will always be an evaluative component to appraise, physician unilateral decision making in the absence of the overwhelming consensus and support of the broader society is never warranted. Physicians might be able to refuse without reproach only when the existence of consensus both within the medical profession, and in the broader society, has been explored and established.

This is not to say that physicians should refrain from decision making until a comprehensive survey of the medical profession is made and society, or some entity representing it, considers the particular details of each and every case. I fully anticipate that standards will be developed and precedents set to establish and support guidelines for decision making in the areas in which we have consensus. The point is that the agreed upon limits will be precisely that—agreed upon, not simply imposed on society by an individual physician or the medical profession at large.

Physicians might begin by using consensus in the medical profession to gauge the likelihood of consensus in the broader community. But without actual consensus and endorsement from the broader community, the medical profession would not be authorized to impose its own conception of appropriate limits. In the absence of consensus and public policy, an individual physician has no more claim to authority than an individual patient. As long as there is controversy, the physician's knowledge claim cannot be sustained, much less defended. Attempts to use judgments of futility, particularly judgments of physiologic futility, are especially problematic because they assert an indefensible knowledge claim of uncontested and uncontestable certainty.

A forum for discussion and review provides the necessary opportunity to challenge such claims, and therefore to contest the physician's authority to impose his judgment on a resisting or unwitting patient. For such a forum, I recommend ethics committees first, and arbitration and the court system as a last resort. I will describe each recommendation in turn.

The Ethics Committee as a Forum and Advisory Body

Ethics committees provide an ideal forum for the consideration of cases of intractable conflict. Multidisciplinary in composition and deliberately designed to be only advisory in nature, they offer a safe and conducive environment for the resolution of difficult cases. The most important task of an ethics committee in a conflict over futility would be to enable all involved parties to express their opinions and concerns. Additionally, the ethics committee would create the opportunity for raising all of the critical questions that have been the focus of this book.

The ethics committee would help establish the source and nature of the conflict between the physician and the patient. If the conflict were over evaluative futility, the ethics committee would consider the prerogative of the patient to make assessments independently, in the absence of any predetermined limits set on social justice grounds and encoded in public policy. The physician's arguments grounded in autonomy, integrity, and moral belief would also be investigated and considered.

If the conflict were over physiologic or factual futility, the ethics committee would help identify the evaluative components of the knowledge claim, considering the strength of the claim and the consensus surrounding it in the medical profession and the broader society. Any pertinent consensually agreed upon guidelines would be presented and considered.

Finally, the ethics committee would offer a non-binding recommendation that would either confirm or reject the physician's arguments for refusing to provide the contested treatment. Of course, another physician might always express a willingness to take over care of the patient, if the bioethics committee recommended against the physician's proposal of treatment refusal. In the end, one of the most important contributions an ethics committee can make is broadening the scope of accountability and insisting on a public defense of the individual physician's or the medical profession's knowledge claim of treatment futility.

The Role of the Courts

Another alternative is to refer all cases of intractable conflict to the courts for resolution in the public domain. The clear advantage of such an approach is that it would include a level of public accountability otherwise absent from either individual physician or individual patient decision making. Such accountability would begin to neutralize the unequal distribution of power and authority in the physician-patient relationship by giving parties an opportunity to present and defend their positions on an equal footing.

Court resolution would also confirm that at issue in these cases are questions resolved most appropriately in the public domain, rather than in the confines of a single physician-patient relationship. In addition, it might create a more consistent approach to such dilemmas, correcting for what might otherwise be a highly variable and idiosyncratic approach to the problem.

Furthermore, court resolution might help focus public discussion and perhaps even lead to consensus about how such dilemmas should be handled in the future. Bringing cases to the court system might arouse public interest and ultimately provide the impetus to change our public policies and laws. The courts have often reminded us that if we do not like the law, we are free to try to change it. This redirection of our attention puts the burden for setting the standards back where it properly belongs—on all of us collectively, rather than on individual physicians or the medical profession. Finally, the court system reflects to some degree existing consensus encoded in the form of statutes, case law, et cetera. So, in some circumstances, a court order might serve as a rough representation of current social consensus.

Of course, resolution by means of the judicial system is not without its problems. One might ask on what grounds and with what warrant a court could better resolve conflicts than the involved care providers, patients, families, and hospital administrators. One might question as a practical matter whether the judicial system is equipped to respond in a timely fashion to such cases. And one might argue that the law and the adversarial legal system are poor instruments for the resolution of complex ethical dilemmas. Nevertheless, I maintain that the court system offers a legitimate, viable solution in cases of intractable conflict.

Summary

In the final analysis, I argue that my alternative recommendations are all superior to the proposal of physician unilateral decision making on the basis of futility. To review, I call first for an investigation of alternative grounds for physician refusal. Next, I call for broad, inclusive, and democratic public discourse and for the development of public policy in response to the issues at stake in the futility debate. I call further for a commitment to genuine conversation featuring complete sentences, moral suasion, and transparent disclosure, especially in the absence of public consensus. And finally, I offer two options for the resolution of any remaining intractable conflicts. Together these recommendations comprise a far more comprehensive and defensible response to the problem of futility than physician unilateral decision making.

It has been my argument that physician unilateral decision making on the basis of futility is a problematic and misguided approach to the challenge of setting appropriate limits in medicine. The futility debate has introduced language, concepts, proposals, and practices that have too narrowly framed possible responses, in either the clinical setting or in public policy, to the paradigmatic conflict between a physician who deems a particular treatment course to be inappropriate and a patient who disagrees and wants the treatment. Moreover, the debate has distracted our collective attention from concerns underlying this conflict between physicians and patients. The ethical dilemma that has given rise to the futility debate is a real one that cannot be simply resolved by naming treatments futile and deciding then that by definition they need not be offered, provided, or continued. In our search for a simple, neat solution to the problem, we have mistakenly turned to the concept of futility. But the concept of futility cannot do what its proponents would have it do. And, in fact, the concept has obscured other considerations in need of our attention.

My goal has not been to offer "the" definitive solution to conflicts over futility, but rather to call for a reframing of the very discussion of and approach to the problem. Once the concept of futility has been rejected, we will be forced to speak and argue in more precise, forthright language about the moral appeals at stake in such conflicts between patients and their care providers. By rejecting the language of futility, I hope to have cleared the way for the important work that remains to be done in addressing and analyzing this complex ethical dilemma. Futility is not the solution; it has only served as an unfortunate distraction. It is time now to direct our attention elsewhere.

NOTES

Chapter One. Whose Facts, Whose Values?

1. David A. Asch, John Hansen-Flaschen, and Paul Lanken, "Decisions to Limit or Continue Life-Sustaining Treatment by Critical Care Physicians in the United States: Conflicts between Physicians' Practices and Patients' Wishes," *American Journal of Respiratory and Critical Care Medicine* 151 (February 1995): 288–92. In this survey of ICU physicians across the country, 83% reported unilaterally withholding and 82% unilaterally withdrawing life sustaining treatment that they judged to be futile.

2. Howard Brody, *The Healer's Power* (New Haven: Yale University Press, 1992); Lawrence J. Schneiderman and Nancy S. Jecker, *Wrong Medicine: Doctors, Patients, and Futile Treatment* (Baltimore: Johns Hopkins University Press, 1995).

3. Representative examples of related uses of the term futility can be found in Lawrence J. Schneiderman, Nancy S. Jecker, and Albert R. Jonsen, "Medical Futility: Its Meaning and Ethical Implications," *Annals of Internal Medicine* 15 (June 15, 1990): 949–54; Schneiderman and Jecker, *Wrong Medicine*; John D. Lantos et al., "The Illusion of Futility in Clinical Practice," *American Journal of Medicine* 87 (July 1989): 81–84; and Robert M. Veatch and Carol Mason Spicer, "Medically Futile Care: The Role of the Physician in Setting Limits," *American Journal of Law and Medicine* 18 (1992): 15–36. The first two use the term quantitative futility to describe outcomes that have a low probability of success and qualitative futility to describe outcomes that have an outcome below a minimum level of acceptability. The third suggests that futile therapies are merely the end of the spectrum of therapies with very low efficacy. The fourth identifies the two types of futile treatment at each end of the spectrum as treatment that produces no demonstrable effect, which is called physiological futility, and treatment that produces an effect that is of no net benefit, which is called normative futility. Veatch and Mason Spicer departed from other commentators on futility by arguing that even judgments of physiological futility necessarily involve conceptual and evaluative judgments (because all purportedly scientific statements do). Schneiderman and Jecker, in their book, as well as others such as Howard Brody and Tom L. Tomlinson, took up this issue later. In Chapter 4, I adopt and expand the general line of argumentation begun by Veatch and Mason Spicer.

4. Schneiderman and Jecker, *Wrong Medicine*.

5. Veatch and Mason Spicer, for example, argue that it is perfectly legitimate

for an equitable funding system to limit or exclude particular treatments. Cf. Veatch and Mason Spicer, "Medically Futile Care."

6. Lantos et al. noted and questioned this tendency to use futility claims to justify radical shifts in physician obligation. See "The Illusion of Futility."

7. The Hastings Center, *Guidelines on the Termination of Life-Sustaining Treatment and the Care of the Dying* (Briarcliff Manor, New York: The Hastings Center, 1987): 32.

8. Stuart Youngner, "Who Defines Futility?" *Journal of the American Medical Association* 260 (October 14, 1988): 2094–95, emphasis added.

9. Allan S. Brett and Laurence B. McCullough, "When Patients Request Specific Interventions: Defining the Limits of the Physician's Obligation," *New England Journal of Medicine* 315 (November 20, 1986): 1349.

10. Schneiderman and Jecker, *Wrong Medicine*.

11. Differentiating the two approaches in this helpful way was suggested to me by Leigh S. Raymond.

12. For some exceptions to this trend, see Brody, *The Healer's Power*; and Schneiderman and Jecker, *Wrong Medicine*. Though increasing attention has been given to such questions in these and other works, I would argue that both the extent of rigorous philosophical analysis and focussed exploration of the normative implications for the futility debate have been insufficient.

13. Plato, *Republic*, Book 3, 407c–e.

14. Ibid., 408a–b.

15. Hippocrates, "The Art," in *Hippocrates*, vol. 2, trans. W. H. S. Jones, Loeb Classical Library (Cambridge: Harvard University Press, 1967): 193.

16. Ibid., 203, 205.

17. This framework addresses treatment decision making between individual patients and their physicians. As such, the emphasis has been on autonomy, beneficence, and nonmaleficence. Respect for the principle of justice might challenge the scope of decision making ultimately available to patients, an issue which I take up later.

18. A. Edward Doudera and J. Douglas Peters, eds., *Legal and Ethical Aspects of Treating Critically and Terminally Ill Patients* (Ann Arbor: AUPHA Press, 1982); President's Commission for the Study of Ethical Problems in Medicine and Biomedical and Behavioral Research, *Deciding to Forego Life Sustaining Treatment: A Report on the Ethical, Medical, and Legal Issues in Treatment Decisions* (Washington, D.C.: U.S. Government Printing Office, March 1983); The President's Commission for the Study of Ethical Problems in Medicine and Biomedical and Behavioral Research, *Making Health Care Decisions: A Report on the Ethical and Legal Implications of Informed Consent in the Patient-Practitioner Relationship* (Washington, D.C.: U.S. Government Printing Office, October 1982); The Hastings Center, *Guidelines*.

19. "Standards and Guidelines for Cardiopulmonary Resuscitation (CPR) and Emergency Cardiac Care (ECC)," supplement, *Journal of the American Medical Association* 227 (February 18, 1974): 864.

20. "Standards and Guidelines for Cardiopulmonary Resuscitation and Emer-

gency Cardiac Care," *Journal of the American Medical Association* 255 (June 6, 1986): 2980.

21. "Ethical Considerations in Resuscitation," *Journal of the American Medical Association* 268 (October 28, 1992): 2282–83.

22. American College of Physicians Ethics Manual, Part 2: "The Physician and Society; Research; Life-Sustaining Treatment; Other Issues," *Annals of Internal Medicine* 111 (August 15, 1989): 333.

23. *American College of Physicians Ethics Manual,* 3rd ed. (U.S.A.: American College of Physicians, 1993): 19.

24. American College of Chest Physicians/Society for Critical Care Medicine (ACCP/SCCM) Consensus Panel, "Ethical and Moral Guidelines for the Initiation, Continuation, and Withdrawal of Intensive Care," *Chest* 97 (April 1990): 951–52.

25. Ibid., 952.

26. American Thoracic Society, Medical Section of the American Lung Association, "Withholding and Withdrawing Life-Sustaining Therapy," *American Review of Respiratory Disease* 144 (September 1991): 728.

27. Council on Ethical and Judicial Affairs, "Guidelines for the Appropriate Use of Do-Not-Resuscitate Orders," *Journal of the American Medical Association* 265 (April 10, 1991): 1870, emphasis added.

28. Council on Ethical and Judicial Affairs, *Code of Medical Ethics* (Chicago: American Medical Association, 1994): 52–53.

29. Ibid., 7.

30. Ibid., 6.

31. "Hospitals Establish Policies to Limit Futile Care," *Hospital Ethics* 9 (September/October 1993): 10–12; Teresa Hudson, "Are Futile-Care Policies the Answer?" *Hospitals and Health Networks* 68 (February 20, 1994): 26–32; Jeremy Sugarman, guest editor, "A Community Policy on Medical Futility? A Conversation of the North Carolina Community," special issue, *North Carolina Medical Journal* 56 (September 1995): 411–72; Tom L. Tomlinson and Diane Czlonka, "Futility and Hospital Policy," *Hastings Center Report* 25 (May/June 1995): 28–35; Donald J. Murphy, "Can We Set Futile Care Policies? Institutional and Systemic Challenges," *Journal of the American Geriatrics Society* 42 (August 1994): 890–93.

32. "Hospitals Establish Policies to Limit Futile Care"; Santa Monica Hospital Medical Center, "Futile Care Guidelines," supplement, *Medical Ethics Advisor* 9 (October 1993); Hudson, "Are Futile-Care Policies the Answer?"

33. "The Johns Hopkins Hospital Policy on Withholding or Withdrawing Futile Life-Sustaining Medical Interventions," (Baltimore: Johns Hopkins Hospital, January 28, 1992), cited in David B. Waisel and Robert D. Troug, "The Cardiopulmonary Resuscitation-Not-Indicated Order: Futility Revisited," *Annals of Internal Medicine* 122 (February 15, 1995): 306.

34. Stewart Shankel, chairman, Futile Care Ad Hoc Committee, San Bernardino County Medical Society, written communication to all area hospital ethics committee chairpersons, April 19, 1995; Eileen S. Lemmon, co-chair, Medical Legal Committee, San Bernardino Medical Society/Bar Association, personal correspondence,

April 2, 1998, and "Optimal Care Proposal," submitted by Medical Legal Committee Optimal Care Task Force, San Bernardino County Medical Society and Bar Association, spring 1998.

35. Donald J. Murphy and Elizabeth Barbour, "GUIDe (Guidelines for the Use of Intensive Care in Denver): A Community Effort to Define Futile and Inappropriate Treatment," *New Horizons* 2 (August 1994): 326–31.

36. Amir Halevy and Baruch A. Brody, "A Multi-institutional Collaborative Policy on Medical Futility," *Journal of the American Medical Association* 276 (August 21, 1996): 571–74.

37. Tomlinson and Czlonka, "Futility and Hospital Policy," 29.

38. "Consensus Statement of the Society of Critical Care Medicine's Ethics Committee Regarding Futile and Other Possibly Inadvisable Treatment," *Critical Care Medicine* 25 (May 1997): 887.

39. *Barber v. Superior Court of California*, 147 Cal. App. 3d 1006, 1017–18, 195 Cal. Rptr. 484 (1983).

40. John J. Paris, Robert K. Crone, and Frank E. Reardon, "Physicians' Refusal of Requested Treatment: The Case of Baby L," *New England Journal of Medicine* 322 (April 5, 1990): 1012–15.

41. Memorandum Issued with Findings of Fact, Conclusions of Law and Order Dated 28 June 1991, *In Re The Conservatorship of Helga M. Wanglie*, # PX-91-283 (District Court Probate Court Division, County of Hennepin, State of Minnesota).

42. *In Re Baby K*, 832 F. Supp. 1022 (E.D. Va. 1993), *aff'd*, 16 F. 3d 590, (4th Cir. 1994) 16 F.3d 590, *cert. denied*, 115 S. Ct. 91, 63 U.S.L.W. 3258, 130 L. Ed. 2d 42 (1994).

43. *In Re Baby K*, 16 F.3d 590 (4th Cir. 1994): 13–14.

44. Gina Kolata, "Withholding Care From Patients: Boston Case Asks, Who Decides?" *New York Times* (April 3, 1995): A1, C10; Kolata, "Court Ruling Limits Rights of Patients: Care Deemed Futile May Be Withheld," *New York Times* (April 22, 1995): A6. *Gilgunn v. Massachusetts General Hospital*, No. 92–4820 (Mass. Sup. Ct. Civ. Action Suffolk Co. April 22, 1995).

45. Ann Dudley Goldlatt, Steven Miles, and others reported the weaning on the Medical College of Wisconsin Internet Bioethics Discussion Forum in May 1995.

46. Interestingly, Donald McNamee, attorney for Catherine Gilgunn's daughter, was also the guardian ad litem in the *Baby L* case.

47. U.S. Department of Health and Human Services, Office of Human Development Services, "Child Abuse and Neglect Prevention and Treatment," *Federal Register* 50 (April 15, 1985): 14878.

48. See, for example, "The Proposed Legislation," app. A in The New York State Task Force on Life and the Law, *Do Not Resuscitate Orders*, 2nd ed. (New York, 1986); "The Virginia Health Care Decisions Act," Virginia Code, Article 8, 54.1-2990.

49. Sharon H. Imbus and Bruce E. Zawacki, "Autonomy for Burned Patients When Survival Is Unprecedented," *New England Journal of Medicine* 297 (August 11, 1977): 308–11.

50. President's Commission, *Deciding to Forego*, 82–90.

51. Pope Pius XII, "The Prolongation of Life: An Address of Pope Pius XII to an International Congress of Anesthesiologists," *The Pope Speaks* 4 (Spring 1958): 395.

52. Ibid., 395.

53. That the preferred perspective is a subjective one does not imply that burden to others is excluded from consideration. In fact, the Pope explicitly recognizes burden to self as well as burden to others as potential factors in a patient's assessment. The important point is that it is up to the patient to consider and weigh the importance of burden to self and others.

54. Congregation for the Doctrine of the Faith, *Declaration On Euthanasia* (Rome: Sacred Congregation for the Doctrine of the Faith, May 5, 1980): 515.

55. Again, emphasis here is on the patient's determination of a treatment's appropriateness, but not necessarily to the exclusion of the patient's determinations about the treatment's effect on others, such as family, the health care team, or the larger society.

56. Congregation for the Doctrine of the Faith, *Declaration On Euthanasia*: 515, emphasis added.

57. Robert M. Veatch, "The Generalization of Expertise: Scientific Expertise and Value Judgments," *The Hastings Center Studies* 1 (1973): 29–40.

58. In Chapter 3, I consider critiques of the generalization of expertise argument that have been offered by Edmund D. Pellegrino, Leon R. Kass, Tomlinson, and Howard Brody. These authors and others have argued that embedded in the medical profession is the self-conscious awareness that its enterprise is a value-rich and inescapably moral one, and that to strip medicine of its values is to mistakenly strip away its essence.

59. Paul S. Applebaum, Charles W. Lidz, and Alan Meisel, *Informed Consent: Legal Theory and Clinical Practice* (New York: Oxford University Press, 1987); Gerald Dworkin, *The Theory and Practice of Autonomy* (Cambridge: Cambridge University Press, 1988); Ruth Faden and Tom Beauchamp, *A History and Theory of Informed Consent* (New York: Oxford University Press, 1986); Robert F. Weir, *Abating Treatment With Critically Ill Patients* (New York: Oxford University Press, 1989).

60. Brett and McCullough, "When Patients Request Specific Interventions"; Brody, *The Healer's Power*; Edmund D. Pellegrino and David C. Thomasma, *For the Patient's Good: The Restoration of Beneficence in Health Care* (New York: Oxford University Press, 1988); Schneiderman and Jecker, *Wrong Medicine*; Lawrence J. Schneiderman, Kathy Faber-Langendoen, and Nancy S. Jecker, "Beyond Futility to an Ethic of Care," *American Journal of Medicine* 96 (February 1994): 110–14; Schneiderman, Jecker, and Jonsen, "Medical Futility; Tom L. Tomlinson and Howard Brody, "Ethics and Communication in Do-Not-Resuscitate Orders," *New England Journal of Medicine* 318 (January 7, 1988): 43–46; Tom L. Tomlinson and Howard Brody, "Futility and the Ethics of Resuscitation," *Journal of the American Medical Association* 264 (September 12, 1990): 1276–80.

61. E. Haavi Morreim, *Balancing Act: The New Medical Ethics of Meidicine's New Economics* (Washington, D.C.: Georgetown University Press, 1995); Marc A. Rodwin, *Medicine, Money, and Morals: Physicians' Conflicts of Interest* (New York: Oxford University Press, 1993.)

62. John D. Lantos, "Futility Assessments and the Doctor-Patient Relationship," *Journal of the American Geriatrics Society* 42 (August 1994): 869.

63. Daniel Y. Chu, "Predicting Survival in AIDS Patients with Respiratory Failure: Application of the APACHE-II Scoring System," *Critical Care Clinics* 9 (January 1993): 89–105; Jack E. Dobkin and Ralph E. Cutler, "Use of APACHE-II Classification to Evaluate Outcomes of Patients Receiving Hemodialysis in an Intensive Care Unit," *Western Journal of Medicine* 149 (November 1988): 547–50; "Futility: Using SUPPORT to GUIDe Our Fix on Futility," *Hospital Ethics* 11 (January/February 1995): 1–5; William A. Knaus et al., "The SUPPORT Prognostic Model: Objective Estimates of Survival for Seriously Ill Hospitalized Adults," *Annals of Internal Medicine* 122 (February 1995): 191–203; William A. Knaus and David B. Nash, "Predicting and Evaluating Patient Outcomes," *Annals of Internal Medicine* 109 (October 1988): 521–22; William A. Knaus et al., "The APACHE III Prognostic System: Risk Prediction of Hospital Mortality for Critically Ill Hospitalized Adults," *Chest* 100 (December 1991): 1619–36; Joanne Lynn and David DeGrazia, "An Outcomes Model of Medical Decision Making," *Theoretical Medicine* 12 (December 1991): 325–43; Joan M. Teno, Donald J. Murphy, Joanne Lynn et al., "Prognosis-Based Futility Guidelines: Does Anyone Win?" *Journal of the American Geriatrics Society* 42 (November 1994): 1202–07; Linda Johnson White, "Clinical Uncertainty, Medical Futility and Practice Guidelines," *Journal of the American Geriatrics Society* 42 (August 1994): 899–901.

64. Cf. Brett and McCullough, "When Patients Request Specific Interventions"; Howard Brody, "The Physician's Role in Determining Futility," *Journal of the American Geriatrics Society* 42 (August 1994): 875–78; Nancy S. Jecker, "Knowing When to Stop: The Limits of Medicine," *Hastings Center Report* 21 (May/June 1991): 5–8; Nancy S. Jecker and Robert A. Pearlman, "Medical Futility: Who Decides?" *Archives of Internal Medicine* 152 (June 1992): 1140–44; Bernard Lo and Albert R. Jonsen, "Clinical Decisions to Limit Treatment," *Annals of Internal Medicine* 93 (November 1980): 764–68; Frank H. Marsh and Allen Staver, "Physician Authority for Unilateral DNR Orders," *Journal of Legal Medicine* 12 (June 1991): 115–65; Paris, Crone, and Reardon, "Physicians' Refusal of Requested Treatment"; Lawrence J. Schneiderman, "The Futility Debate: Effective versus Beneficial Intervention," *Journal of the American Geriatrics Society* 42 (August 1994): 883–86; Schneiderman, Faber-Langendoen, and Jecker, "Beyond Futility to an Ethic of Care"; Schneiderman and Jecker, *Wrong Medicine*; Schneiderman, Jecker, and Jonsen, "Medical Futility"; Lawrence J. Schneiderman, Nancy S. Jecker, and Albert R. Jonsen, "Medical Futility: Response to Critiques," *Annals of Internal Medicine* 125 (October 15, 1996): 669–74; Tomlinson and Brody, "Ethics and Communication"; Tomlinson and Brody, "Futility and the Ethics of Resuscitation."

65. Cf. Felicia Ackerman, "The Significance of a Wish," *Hastings Center Report* 21 (July/August 1991): 27–29; Ann Alpers and Bernard Lo, "Futility: Not Just a Medical Issue," *Law, Medicine, and Health Care* 20 (Winter 1992): 327–29; Troyen A. Brennan, "Silent Decisions: Limits of Consent and the Terminally Ill Patient," *Law, Medicine, and Health Care* 16 (Fall/Winter 1988): 204–9; Baruch A. Brody and Amir Halevy, "Is Futility a Futile Concept?" *Journal of Medicine and Philosophy* 20 (April 1995): 123–44; Daniel Callahan, "Medical Futility, Medical Necessity: The-Problem-Without-A-Name," *Hastings Center Report* 21 (July/August 1991): 30–35; Lantos, "Futility Assessments and the Doctor-Patient Relationship"; Lantos et al., "The Illu-

sion of Futility"; Thomas J. Prendergast, "Futility and the Common Cold: How Requests for Antibiotics Can Illuminate Care at the End of Life," *Chest* 107 (March 1995): 836–44; Mildred Z. Solomon, "How Physicians Talk about Futility: Making Words Mean Too Many Things," *Law, Medicine, and Ethics* 21 (Summer 1993): 231–37; Rosemarie Tong, "Towards a Just, Courageous, and Honest Resolution of the Futility Debate," *Journal of Medicine and Philosophy* 20 (April 1995): 165–89; Robert T. Troug, "Beyond Futility," *Journal of Clinical Ethics* 3 (Summer 1992): 143–45; Robert T. Troug, Allan S. Brett, and Joel Frader, "The Problem With Futility," *New England Journal of Medicine* 326 (June 4, 1992): 1560–64; Robert M. Veatch, "Why Physicians Cannot Determine If Care Is Futile," *Journal of the American Geriatrics Society* 42 (August 1994): 871–74; Veatch and Mason Spicer, "Medically Futile Care"; Susan M. Wolf, "Conflict Between Doctor and Patient," *Law, Medicine, and Health Care* 16 (Fall/Winter 1988): 197–203; Youngner, "Who Defines Futility?" Stuart J. Youngner, "Futility in Context," *Journal of the American Medical Association* 264 (September 12, 1990): 1295–96.

Chapter Two. What Do People Mean by Futility?

1. *Oxford English Dictionary* and *The Concise Oxford Dictionary of English Etymology.*

2. Schneiderman, Jecker, and Jonsen, "Medical Futility," 950.

3. Schneiderman and Jecker, *Wrong Medicine*, 19.

4. Consider, for example, our changing notions of effective and appropriate treatment for premature infants with respiratory distress or for pregnant women with anxiety or depression. Treatments that were once recommended routinely are now regarded as harmful.

5. I take up the concept of relevance more directly in Chapter 5.

6. Youngner, "Who Defines Futility?" 2094. Youngner expands upon this point in "Applying Futility: Saying No Is Not Enough," *Journal of the American Geriatrics Society* 42 (August 1994): 887–89.

7. This helpful grammatical analogue was suggested to me by Esther Wagner.

8. David Feldman, *Health and Medicine in the Jewish Tradition* (New York: Crossroad Publishing, National Conference, 1986); "Standards and Guidelines for (CPR) and (ECC)," 1974; Youngner, "Who Defines Futility?" 2094.

9. Youngner, "Who Defines Futility?" 2094.

10. Tomlinson and Brody, "Ethics and Communication," 43; Youngner, "Who Defines Futility?" 2094.

11. Brett and McCullough, "When Patients Request Specific Interventions"; Gerald Kelly, *Medico Moral Problems* (St. Louis: Catholic Hospital Association, 1958): 135; Tomlinson and Brody, "Ethics and Communication," 43.

12. Schneiderman, Jecker, and Jonsen, "Medical Futility," 950.

13. *Barber v. Superior Court of California.*

14. Schneiderman, Jecker, and Jonsen, "Medical Futility," 950; Schneiderman and Jecker, *Wrong Medicine* 159; David C. Thomasma, "Beyond Medical Paternalism

and Patient Autonomy: A Model of Physician Conscience for the Physician-Patient Relationship," *Annals of Internal Medicine* 98 (February 1983): 243–48.

15. Lo and Jonsen, "Clinical Decisions to Limit Treatment," 764; Paris, Crone, and Reardon, "Physicians' Refusal of Requested Treatment," 1013.

16. Susan Wolf, qtd. in Lisa Belkin, "As Family Protests," *New York Times*, January 10, 1991: A1, A16.

17. Article 29-B, Statute 413-A, The State of New York Public Health Law, 1988; The New York State Task Force on Life and the Law, *Do Not Resuscitate Orders*.

18. Jecker and Pearlman, "Medical Futility," 1143; 1984 Amendments to the Child Abuse Prevention and Treatment Act, Public Law 98-457, 1984; Schneiderman, Jecker, and Jonsen, "Medical Futility," 950; Schneiderman and Jecker, *Wrong Medicine*, 17.

19. Schneiderman, Jecker, and Jonsen, "Medical Futility," 952–53; Schneiderman and Jecker, *Wrong Medicine*, 17.

20. Lantos et al., "The Illusion of Futility," 81; Lo and Jonsen, "Clinical Decisions to Limit Treatment," 764.

21. Lo and Jonsen, "Clinical Decisions to Limit Treatment," 764.

22. Susanna E. Bedell, et al., "Survival after Cardiopulmonary Resuscitation in the Hospital," *New England Journal of Medicine* 309 (September 8, 1983): 569–76; Leslie J. Blackhall, "Must We Always Use CPR?" *New England Journal of Medicine* 317 (November 12, 1987): 1281–84.

23. George E. Taffet, Thomas A. Teasdale, and Robert J. Luchi, "In-Hospital Cardiopulmonary Resuscitation," *Journal of the American Medical Association* 260 (October 14, 1988): 2069–72.

24. Henry S. Perkins, "Ethics at the End of Life: Practical Principles for Making Resuscitation Decisions," *Journal of General Internal Medicine* 1 (May/June 1986): 170–76; John E. Ruark and Thomas A. Raffin, "Initiating and Withdrawing Life Support: Principles and Practice in Adult Medicine," *New England Journal of Medicine* 318 (January 7, 1988): 25–30.

25. Jecker and Pearlman, "Medical Futility," Schneiderman, Jecker, and Jonsen, "Medical Futility," 951–52; Youngner, "Who Defines Futility?" 2094.

26. Schneiderman and Jecker, *Wrong Medicine*, 129.

27. Tomlinson and Czlonka, "Futility and Hospital Policy," 32.

28. Robert D. Troug, "Progress in the Futility Debate," *Journal of Clinical Ethics* 6 (Summer 1995): 129.

29. Schneiderman and Jecker, *Wrong Medicine*, 153–54.

30. Ibid., 5.

31. Robert A. Pearlman and Albert R. Jonsen, "The Use of Quality-of-Life Considerations in Medical Decision Making," *Journal of the American Geriatrics Society* 33 (May 1985): 344–52.

32. I have learned much about the limits of our ability to judge quality of life in discussions with my colleague, Laurie Zoloth-Dorfman. Rather than presuming we can have access to a patient's quality of life, Zoloth-Dorfman suggests we limit our description to an account of that portion of a patient's daily life that is exposed to the external world and therefore to our perceptions.

33. Marion Danis et al., "Patients' and Families' Preferences for Medical Intensive Care," *Journal of the American Medical Association* 260 (August 12, 1988): 797–802; Robert A. Pearlman, Richard F. Uhlmann, and Nancy S. Jecker, "Spousal Understanding of Patient Quality of Life: Implications for Surrogate Decision Making," *Journal of Clinical Ethics* 3 (Summer 1992): 114–120; Lawrence J. Schneiderman et al., "Do Physicians' Own Preferences for Life-Sustaining Treatment Influence Their Perceptions of Patients' Preferences?" *Journal of Clinical Ethics* 4 (Spring 1993): 28–32; Richard F. Uhlmann, Robert A. Pearlman, and Kevin C. Cain, "Physicians' and Spouses' Predictions of Elderly Patients' Resuscitation Preferences," *Journal of Gerontology* 43 (September 1988): M115–21.

34. *In Re Quinlan*, 70 N.J. 10, 355 A.2d 647, cert. denied sub nom. *Garger v. New Jersey*, 429 U.S. 922 (1976).

35. Richard A. McCormick, S.J., *Notes on Moral Theology: 1965–1980* (Lanham, Maryland: University Press of America, 1981).

36. Jecker and Pearlman, "Medical Futility," 1143.

37. Memorandum, *In Re The Conservatorship of Helga M. Wanglie.*

38. Donald J. Murphy et al., "Outcomes of Cardiopulmonary Resuscitation in the Elderly," *Annals of Internal Medicine* 111 (August 1, 1989): 199; Taffet et al., "In-Hospital Cardiopulmonary Resuscitation."

39. Bedell et al., "Survival after Cardiopulmonary Resuscitation in the Hospital"; Murphy, et al., "Outcomes of Cardiopulmonary Resuscitation in the Elderly."

40. Bedell et al., "Survival after Cardiopulmonary Resuscitation in the Hospital."

41. Bedell et al., "Survival after Cardiopulmonary Resuscitation in the Hospital"; Kathy Faber-Langendoen, "Resuscitation of Patients With Metastatic Cancer: Is Transient Benefit Still Futile?" *Archives of Internal Medicine* 151 (February 1991): 235–39; Taffet et al., "In-Hospital Cardiopulmonary Resuscitation."

42. Taffet et al., "In-Hospital Cardiopulmonary Resuscitation."

43. John D. Lantos et al., "Survival After Cardiopulmonary Resuscitation in Babies of Very Low Birth Weight: Is CPR Futile Therapy?" *New England Journal of Medicine* 318 (January 14, 1988): 91–95.

44. William A. Gray, Robert J. Capone, and Albert S. Most, "Unsuccessful Emergency Medical Resuscitation—Are Continued Efforts in the Emergency Department Justified?" *New England Journal of Medicine* 325 (November 14, 1991): 1393–98.

45. Schneiderman, Jecker, and Jonsen, "Medical Futility"; Schneiderman and Jecker, *Wrong Medicine.*

46. Brennan, "Silent Decisions"; Imbus and Zawacki, "Autonomy for Burned Patients"; Lantos et al., "The Illusion of Futility," 83; Tomlinson and Brody, "Ethics and Communication," 44; Truog, Brett, and Frader, "The Problem With Futility," 1561; Youngner, "Who Defines Futility?"

47. Albert R. Jonsen, "Do No Harm," *Annals of Internal Medicine* 88 (June 1978): 829.

48. Charles Fried, *Anatomy of Values* (Cambridge: Harvard University Press, 1970): 177.

49. Brett and McCullough, "When Patients Request Specific Interventions"; Marsh and Staver, "Physician Authority"; Paris, Crone, and Reardon, "Physicians'

Refusal of Requested Treatment"; Edmund D. Pellegrino, "Withholding and With-drawing Treatments: Ethics at the Bedside," *Clinical-Neurosurgery* 35 (1989): 164–84; Schneiderman, Jecker, and Jonsen, "Medical Futility."

50. Schneiderman, Jecker, and Jonsen, "Medical Futility," 951.

51. Jecker and Pearlman, "Medical Futility," 1140.

52. Molly L. Osborne, "Physician Decisions Regarding Life Support in the In-tensive Care Unit," *Chest* 101 (January 1992): 222–23.

53. Veatch and Mason Spicer, "Medically Futile Care."

54. Jecker and Pearlman, "Medical Futility," 1142–43.

55. Robert M. Veatch, "Consensus of Expertise: The Role of Consensus of Ex-perts in Formulating Public Policy and Estimating Facts," *Journal of Medicine and Philosophy* 16 (August 1991): 427–45.

56. Kathryn Montgomery Hunter, "There Was This One Guy. . . . : The Uses of Anecdotes in Medicine," *Perspectives in Biology and Medicine* 29 (Summer 1986): 619–30.

57. Gina Kolata, "Heart Study Reports Early Revival Is Key to Surviving Attack," *New York Times*, November 14, 1991: A1, A11.

58. Gray, Capone, and Most, "Unsuccessful Emergency Medical Resuscitation."

59. Of course, it is also necessary to note that all statistical data is collected and analyzed with a particular confidence interval, or level of potential error. So the re-port of the cardiologist who knew of a patient who had lived might be understood not as contradicting the data, but as falling within the range of the confidence in-terval.

60. George M. Brockway, "The Physician's Appeal to Firsthand Experience," *Hastings Center Report* 6 (April 1976): 9–12; Alvan R. Feinstein, *Clinical Judgment* (Baltimore: Williams and Wilkins, 1967).

61. Mary E. Charlson et al., "Assessing Illness Severity: Does Clinical Judgment Work?" *Journal of Chronic Diseases* 39 (June 1986): 439–52.

62. John M. Eisenberg, "Sociologic Influences on Decision-Making by Clini-cians," *Annals of Internal Medicine* 90 (June 1979): 957–64.

63. Robert M. Wachter et al., "Decisions about Resuscitation: Inequities among Patients with Different Diseases But Similar Prognoses," *Annals of Internal Medicine* 111 (September 1989): 525–32.

64. Schneiderman, Jecker, and Jonsen, "Medical Futility," 951.

65. Arnold S. Relman, "Assessment and Accountability: The Third Revolution in Medical Care," *New England Journal of Medicine* 319 (November 3, 1988): 1220–22.

66. Arnold M. Epstein, "The Outcomes Movement—Will It Get Us Where We Want to Go?" *New England Journal of Medicine* 323 (July 26, 1990): 267.

67. Ibid., 266.

68. David A. Grimes, "Technological Follies: The Uncritical Acceptance of Medical Innovation," *Journal of the American Medical Association* 269 (June 16, 1993): 3032.

69. William A. Knaus, Douglas P. Wagner, and Joanne Lynn, "Short-Term Mor-tality Predictions for Critically Ill Hospitalized Adults: Science and Ethics," *Science* 254 (October 18, 1991): 390.

70. A more recent development has been the completion of SUPPORT (The Study to Understand Prognoses and Preferences for Outcomes and Risks of Treatment), a multicenter study designed to examine outcomes and clinical decision making for seriously ill hospitalized patients, and to develop and validate a prognostic model that estimates survival over a 180-day period. Cf. Knaus et al., "The SUPPORT Prognostic Model."

71. Knaus, Wagner, and Lynn, "Short-Term Mortality Predictions."

72. Ibid., 392.

73. Jonsen, "Do No Harm," 829.

74. D. Alan Shewmon, "Caution in the Definition and Diagnosis of Infant Brain Death," in *Medical Ethics: A Guide for Health Professionals*, (ed. John F. Monagle and David C. Thomasma) (Maryland: Aspen Press, 1988): 38–57; and D. Alan Shewmon, "Ethics and Brain Death: A Response," *New Scholasticism* 61 (Summer 1987): 321–44.

75. This is an issue that has yet to be resolved. Among the questions still debated are the following. Must the principles be lexically ordered according to an overarching theory, as Robert M. Veatch suggests in *A Theory of Medical Ethics* (New York: Basic Books, 1981)? Should the principles remain unranked as Tom Beauchamp and James F. Childress suggest in *Principles of Biomedical Ethics* (New York: Oxford University Press, 1989)? Should something like reflective equilibrium guide our use of principles and their application to cases, as suggested by John Rawls in *A Theory of Justice* (Cambridge, Massachusetts: Harvard University Press, 1971)?

76. Theories like Veatch's offer some protection against this problem by insisting on a lexical ordering of principles.

77. See, for example, Baruch Brody, *Life and Death Decisionmaking* (New York: Oxford University Press, 1988) and Albert R. Jonsen and Stephen Toulmin, *The Abuse of Casuistry* (Berkeley: University of California Press, 1988).

Chapter Three. A Question of Values

1. Case drawn from my experience as a clinical ethicist.

2. This case, while clearly an example of a physician making an evaluative futility judgment about the worth of a course of treatment, could be modified to encompass a conflict over the facts, as Robert M. Veatch suggested to me. If the physician based his futility judgment on a purportedly factual claim that the patient would not be able to "kick the habit," and he and the patient disagreed not about the worth of breaking the addiction, but rather about the odds of her being able to successfully do so, this case would qualify as a case of conflict over factual futility as well. I consider such cases in Chapter 4.

3. To test the power of prejudice in judgments of evaluative futility, my colleague, Laurie Zoloth-Dorfman, and I have presented this case in conjunction with a clinically identical case that differs only in patient profile. We have found that when the patient is described as an alcoholic, clinicians are remarkably consistent in their tendency to view further treatment as futile. When the patient is described as a likable mother of three who accidentally ate toxic mushrooms at a church picnic,

further treatment, including transplantation, is typically judged to be entirely worthwhile. Clinicians make these judgments despite their knowledge of statistical evidence of alcoholics being transplanted with success.

4. See, for example, Jecker and Pearlman, "Medical Futility"; and Schneiderman, Jecker, and Jonsen, "Medical Futility."

5. I participated in this case consultation with my colleague, Laurie Zoloth-Dorfman. Zoloth-Dorfman has independently reflected on the meaning and significance of this case in her dissertation, *Community and Conscience: The Language of Justice and the Ethics of Health Care Reform* (1993), and in *The Ethics of Encounter*, forthcoming from University of North Carolina Press.

6. Memorandum, *In Re The Conservatorship of Helga M. Wanglie.*

7. Bruce E. Zawacki, M.D., shared this case from his practice with me in a personal conversation in December 1990. I obtained clarification of the case from him through personal correspondence in July 1993.

8. I elaborate further on society's interests and their relationship to patient and physician decisions in Chapter 5.

9. Veatch, "Generalization of Expertise."

10. I leave open the question of whether being in an epistemically privileged position is a necessary condition for decision making authority. The liberal view would argue that patients can claim evaluative authority even if they are not in an epistemically privileged position.

11. Imbus and Zawacki, "Autonomy for Burned Patients," 310.

12. Edmund D. Pellegrino and David C. Thomasma, *A Philosophical Basis of Medical Practice: Toward a Philosophy and Ethic of the Healing Professions* (New York: Oxford University Press, 1981).

13. Leon R. Kass, *Toward a More Natural Science: Biology and Human Affairs* (New York: Free Press, 1985).

14. Tomlinson and Brody, "Futility and the Ethics of Resuscitation."

15. Schneiderman and Jecker, *Wrong Medicine.*

16. Jecker and Pearlman, "Medical Futility."

17. Tomlinson and Brody, "Futility and the Ethics of Resuscitation."

18. Jecker and Pearlman, "Medical Futility," 1140.

19. Tomlinson and Brody, "Futility and the Ethics of Resuscitation," 1279.

20. Schneiderman and Jecker, *Wrong Medicine,* 159.

21. Ibid., 104–5.

22. Ibid., 127.

23. For one of the best treatments of the concept of paternalism, see James F. Childress, *Who Should Decide? Paternalism in Health Care* (New York: Oxford University Press, 1982). I have used Childress's distinctions and analysis in this section on paternalism.

24. I address the relationship of individual want or need and societal obligation in Chapter 5, with particular attention to the obligation society might have to protect the interests of minorities whose values are not reflected in the established priorities of the public.

Chapter Four. The Power of Positivist Thinking

1. My thanks go to Carol Bayley for this provocative and descriptive title.

2. Brody, *The Healer's Power*, 175–76.

3. Ibid., 173–74.

4. "Positivism" has been used to describe a particular philosophical outlook. While a complete theory of positivism cannot be found in any one single repository, some of the clearest statements of positivism, specifically logical positivism or, as it was also called, scientific empiricism, can be traced to the Vienna circle. For representatives of this tradition, see the work of Rudolf Carnap, Herbert Feigl, and Moritz Schlick.

5. Richard Rorty describes this as the ideal of "representing things as they really are" in *Philosophy and the Mirror of Nature* (Princeton: Princeton University Press, 1979): 334.

6. Helen E. Longino, *Science as Social Knowledge: Values and Objectivity in Scientific Inquiry* (Princeton: Princeton University Press, 1990).

7. Bedell, "Survival after Cardiopulmonary Resuscitation"; Leslie J. Blackhall, "Low Survival Rate After Cardiopulmonary Resuscitation in a County Hospital," *Archives of Internal Medicine* 152 (October 1992): 2045–48; Chu, "Predicting Survival"; Richard O. Cummins and Mickey S. Eisenberg, "Prehospital Cardio-pulmonary Resuscitation: Is It Effective?" *Journal of the American Medical Association* 253 (April 26, 1985): 2408–12; Faber-Langendoen, "Resuscitation of Patients with Metastatic Cancer"; Stanley B. Fiel, "Heart-Lung Transplantation for Patients With Cystic Fibrosis: A Test of Clinical Wisdom," *Archives of Internal Medicine* 151 (May 1991): 870–72; Peter A. Gross, "Comparison of Severity of Illness Indicators in an Intensive Care Unit," *Archives of Internal Medicine* 151 (November 1991): 2201–5; Michael P. Hosking et al., "Outcomes of Surgery in Patients 90 Years of Age and Older," *Journal of the American Medical Association* 261 (August 18, 1989): 1909–15; Knaus et al., "The SUPPORT Prognostic Model"; Francis J. Landry, Joseph M. Parker, and Yancy Y. Phillips, "Outcome of Cardiopulmonary Resuscitation in the Intensive Care Setting," *Archives of Internal Medicine* 152 (November 1992): 2305–8; Van S. McCrary et al., "Physicians' Quantitative Assessments of Medical Futility," *Journal of Clinical Ethics* 5 (Summer 1994): 100–5; Donald J. Murphy et al., "Outcomes of Cardiopulmonary Resuscitation in the Elderly"; Daniel P. Schuster and Jay M. Marion, "Precedents for Meaningful Recovery During Treatment in Medical Intensive Care Units: Outcomes in Patients with Hematologic Malignancy," *American Journal of Medicine* 75 (September 1983): 402–8; Martin Urberg and Carol Ways, "Survival After Cardiopulmonary Resuscitation for an In-Hospital Cardiac Arrest," *Journal of Family Practice* 25 (July 1987): 41–44.

8. Mary E. Hawkesworth, "From Objectivity to Objectification," in *Rethinking Objectivity*, ed. Allan Megill (Durham, North Carolina: Duke University Press, 1994): 154.

9. Allan Megill, introduction to *Rethinking Objectivity*, ed. Megill, 1.

10. See for example, Barry Barnes, *Scientific Knowledge and Sociological Theory* (London: Routledge and Kegan Paul, 1974); Mary Hess, *Revolutions and Reconstructions in the Philosophy of Science* (Bloomington: Indiana University Press, 1980); Larry Laudan, *Science and Values* (Berkeley: University of California Press, 1984); Longino, *Science as Social Knowledge*; Steven Shapin, "History of Science and its Sociological Constructions," *History of Science* 20 (1982): 157–211.

11. Terry Eagleton, *Literary Theory* (Oxford: Blackwell Press, 1985); Bruno Latour and Steve Woolgar, *Laboratory Life: The Social Construction of Scientific Facts* (Beverly Hills: Sage, 1979); Greg Meyers, *Writing Biology* (Madison: University of Wisconsin Press, 1990); George Levine, "Why Science Isn't Literature," in Megill, *Rethinking Objectivity*, 65–79.

12. See, for example, Lorraine Code, *What Can She Know? Feminist Theory and the Construction of Knowledge* (Ithaca: Cornell University Press, 1991); Sandra Harding, *The Science Question in Feminism* (Ithaca: Cornell University Press, 1986); Donna Haraway, "Situated Knowledges: The Science Question in Feminism and the Privilege of Partial Perspective," *Feminist Studies* 14 (Fall 1988): 575–99; Alison M. Jaggar and Susan R. Bordo, eds., *Gender/Body/Knowledge: Feminist Reconstructions of Being and Knowing* (New Brunswick: Rutgers University Press, 1989); Evelyn Fox Keller, *Reflections on Gender and Science* (New Haven: Yale University Press, 1985); Liz Stanley and Sue Wise, *Breaking Out: Feminist Consciousness and Feminist Research* (London: Routledge and Kegan Paul, 1983).

13. See Ludwik Fleck, *Genesis and Development of a Scientific Fact* (1935; reprint, Chicago, Illinois: University of Chicago Press, 1979).

14. See Thomas Kuhn, *The Structure of Scientific Revolutions*, 2nd ed. (Chicago, Illinois: University of Chicago Press, 1970).

15. Levine, "Why Science Isn't Literature," 68.

16. Thomas Nagel, *The View from Nowhere* (New York: Oxford University Press, 1986).

17. Levine, "Why Science Isn't Literature," 69.

18. Lorraine Code, "Who Cares?" in Megill, *Rethinking Objectivity*, 181.

19. See Mary E. Hawkesworth, "From Objectivity to Objectification," 154; and Catharine MacKinnon, *Feminism Unmodified* (Cambridge: Harvard University Press, 1987): 50–55.

20. Notable exceptions can be found in Veatch and Mason Spicer, "Medically Futile Care"; and in Robert M. Veatch and William E. Stempsey, "Incommensurability: Its Implications for the Patient/Physician Relationship," *Journal of Medicine and Philosophy* 20 (June 1995): 253–69.

21. Longino, *Science as Social Knowledge*, 83–85.

22. Robert K. Merton, "Science, Technology and Society in Seventeenth-Century England," *Osiris* 4 (1938): 360–62.

23. Longino, *Science as Social Knowledge*, 86.

24. See Robert M. Veatch, *Value-Freedom in Science and Technology* (Missoula, MT: Scholars Press, 1976), especially Chapter 9.

25. Carol Korenbrot, "Experiences with Systemic Contraceptives," *Toxic Sub-*

stances: Decisions and Values, Conference II: Information Flow (Washington, D.C.: Technical Information Project, 1979): 11–42.

26. Gregory Pincus, *The Control of Fertility* (New York: Academic Press, 1965).

27. D. Alan Shewmon, "Caution in the Definition and Diagnosis"; "Commentary on Guidelines for the Determination of Brain Death in Children," Annals of Neurology 24 (December 1988): 789–91; "Ethics and Brain Death."

28. Wendy L. Schoen, note, "Conflict in the Parameters Defining Life and Death in Missouri Statutes," *American Journal of Law and Medicine* 16 (1990): 555–72; Veatch and Mason Spicer, "Medically Futile Care," 19; Robert M. Veatch, *Death, Dying, and the Biological Revolution: Our Last Quest for Responsibility*, rev. ed. (New Haven: Yale University Press, 1989).

29. Mark McClellan, Barbara J. McNeil, and Joseph P. Newhouse, "Does More Intensive Treatment of Acute Myocardial Infarction in the Elderly Reduce Mortality? Analysis Using Instrumental Variables," *Journal of the American Medical Association* 272 (September 21, 1994): 859–66.

30. Brody, *The Healer's Power*, 180.

31. Schneiderman, Jecker, and Jonsen, "Medical Futility: Response to Critiques," 671.

32. Harding, *The Science Question in Feminism*, 36; Elizabeth Fee, "Women's Nature and Scientific Objectivity," in *Women's Nature: Rationalizations of Inequality*, ed. Marian Lowe and Ruth Hubbard (New York: Pergamon, 1983): 16.

33. See Mary Hesse, "Theory and Observation," in Hesse, *Revolutions and Reconstructions in the Philosophy of Science* (Bloomington: Indiana University Press, 1980): 63–110.

34. Francis Bacon, *Novum organum*, cit. n. 1, Bk. 1, Aphorism 46.

35. Longino, *Science as Social Knowledge*, 43.

36. Ibid., 40.

37. Ibid., 43.

38. Using this understanding of background beliefs she offers new interpretations of the Michelson-Morley interferometer experiments in the late nineteenth century and of Priestley's experiments in the late eighteenth century.

39. Schneiderman, Jecker, and Jonsen, "Medical Futility."

40. Schneiderman, Jecker, and Jonsen, "Medical Futility: Response to Critiques," 672.

41. As frequently noted, in Bayesian analysis, unlike standard statistical analysis, the convergence of data from clinical trials on the one hand, and clinical predictions based on prior beliefs and theories on the other hand, decreases the uncertainty otherwise associated with smaller sample sizes. See James M. Brophy and Lawrence Joseph, "Placing Trials in Context Using Bayesian Analysis," *Journal of the American Medical Association* 273 (March 15, 1995): 871–75; Alvan R. Feinstein, "*Clinical Judgment* Revisited: The Distraction of Quantitative Models," *Annals of Internal Medicine* 120 (May 1994): 799–805.

42. Marianne A. Paget, *The Unity of Mistakes: A Phenomenological Interpretation of Medical Work* (Philadelphia: Temple University Press, 1988); see also Paget, *A*

Complex Sorrow, ed. Marjorie L. DeVault (Philadelphia: Temple University Press, 1993), for a moving account of Paget's personal experience with, and ultimate death as a result of, medical error.

43. Charles L. Bosk, *Forgive and Remember: Managing Medical Failure* (Chicago: University of Chicago Press, 1979).

44. Marcia Millman, *The Unkindest Cut: Life in the Backrooms of Medicine* (New York: Morrow Quill, 1977).

45. Lawrence K. Altman, "Antimicrobial Drugs Endorsed for Ulcers in a Major U.S. Shift," *New York Times,* February 10, 1994: A1 and C18.

46. Lawrence K. Altman, "Stomach Microbe Offers Clues to Cancer as Well as Ulcers," *New York Times,* February 22, 1994: B6.

47. In recent history, one can cite numerous examples of radically different scientific and clinical beliefs that have been held over time regarding effective, appropriate, and safe treatments for particular conditions or patient populations. In obstetrics, for example, it would approach heresy today to prescribe a nightly glass of wine to an anxious pregnant woman, but it was commonplace several generations ago. Similarly, it would have been unthinkable to offer vaginal delivery to a woman who had previously had a cesarean section, but today vaginal births after cesarean section (VBAC) are quite common. Similar examples can be cited in every practice area of medicine.

48. *In Re Baby K, aff'd, cert. denied;* "Death of Baby K Leaves a Legacy of Legal Precedents," *The Washington Post* April 7, 1995: B3.

49. Zoloth-Dorfman has reflected independently on this case in her dissertation, *Community and Conscience,* and in her forthcoming book, *The Ethics of Encounter.*

50. A commitment was made to this patient to use his story for educational purposes; he regarded the use of his first name as a way to "live on" through our teaching.

Chapter Five. After Futility

1. Veatch, *A Theory of Medical Ethics.*

2. Veatch and Mason Spicer, "Medically Futile Care," 27.

3. Robert M. Veatch, "What Counts as Basic Health Care? Private Values and Public Policy," *Hastings Center Report* 24 (May/June 1994): 20–21. According to Veatch's interpretation of the contract, until such time as a better pairing of patients and health care providers is possible, along the lines of shared value systems, the medical profession as a whole bears a collective responsibility not to abandon patients, but rather to make treatment available under agreed upon circumstances, even if the particular practitioner disagrees with the course of treatment.

4. Schneiderman and Jecker, *Wrong Medicine,* 153–54.

5. Ibid., 153.

6. Callahan, "Medical Futility, Medical Necessity," 31–32.

7. Jonathon D. Moreno, *Deciding Together: Bioethics and Moral Consensus* (New York: Oxford University Press, 1995).

8. Daniel Yankelovich, *Coming to Public Judgment: Making Democracy Work in a Complex World* (Syracuse: Syracuse University Press, 1991).

9. Charles J. Dougherty, "Setting Health Care Priorities," special supplement, *Hastings Center Report* 21 (May/June 1991): 1–10.

10. Bruce Jennings, "A Grassroots Movement in Bioethics," Special Supplement, *Hastings Center Report* 18 (June/July 1988): 1–16; Jennings et al., "Grassroots Bioethics Revisited: Health Care Priorities and Community Values," special issue, *Hastings Center Report* 20 (September/October 1990): 16–23.

11. Brody, *Healer's Power*, 185.

12. Ibid., 185.

13. Ibid., 184.

14. There is strong legal precedence for considering the maintenance of the integrity of the medical profession to be a compelling state interest. See, for example, *Washington v. Glucksberg*, 138 L. Ed. 2d 772 (1977); *Vacco v. Quill*, 138 L. Ed. 2d 834 (1977); *Bartling v. Superior Court*, 163 Cal. App. 3d 186, 209 Cal. Rptr. 220 (1984); *Superintendent of Belchertown State School v. Saikewicz*, 373 Mass. 728, 370 N.E. 2d 417 (1977).

15. A notable exception to this claim can be found in the work of Dorle Vawter and Karen Gervais at the Minnesota Center for Health Care Ethics. See Vawter, letter to the editor, "The Houston City Wide Policy on Medical Futility," *Journal of the American Medical Association* 276 (November 20, 1996): 1549–50; Vawter, "Professional Integrity Based Objections to Providing Requested Interventions," paper presented at the Ninth Annual Bioethics Summer Retreat, Hilton Head Island, South Carolina, June 11–15, 1997.

16. "Hospitals Establish Policies to Limit Futile Care"; Hudson, "Are Futile-Care Policies the Answer?" Murphy and Barbour, "GUIDe (Guidelines for the Use of Intensive Care Services in Denver)"; Sugarman, "A Community Policy on Medical Futility?" Tomlinson and Czlonka, "Futility and Hospital Policy"; Halevy and Brody, "A Multi-institutional Collaborative Policy."

17. Ralph Crawshaw, Michael Garland, and Brian Hines, "Oregon Health Decisions: An Experiment with Informed Community Consent," *Journal of the American Medical Association* 254 (December 13, 1985): 3213–16; Michael Garland, "Justice, Politics, and Community: Expanding Access and Rationing Health Services in Oregon," *Law, Medicine and Health Care* 20 (Spring/Summer 1992): 67–72.

18. "New Jersey Declaration of Death Act," N.J. Stat. Chs. 26: 6A-1 through 6A-8 (West 1994).

19. Robert S. Olick, "Brain Death, Religious Freedom, and Public Policy: New Jersey's Landmark Legislative Initiative," *Kennedy Institute of Ethics Journal* 1 (December 1991): 275–88.

20. Veatch and Mason Spicer, "Medically Futile Care."

21. Veatch, "What Counts as Basic Health Care?" Robert M. Veatch, "Contemporary Bioethics and the Demise of Modern Medicine," in *The Patient-Physician Relation: The Patient as Partner, Part 2* (Bloomington: Indiana University Press, 1991): 263–79.

22. Stephen G. Post, "My Conscience, Your Money: Commentary," *Hastings Center Report* 25 (September/October 1995): 28.

23. Tomlinson and Brody, "Ethics and Communication." Tomlinson and Brody, "Futility and the Ethics of Resuscitation"; Schneiderman, Faber-Langendoen, and Jecker, "Beyond Futility to an Ethic of Care"; Tomlinson and Czlonka, "Futility and Hospital Policy"; Schneiderman and Jecker, *Wrong Medicine*; Halevy and Brody, "A Multi-institutional Collaborative Policy."

24. Brody, *Healer's Power*, 183, emphasis added.

25. Howard Brody, "Transparency: Informed Consent in Primary Care," *Hastings Center Report* 19 (September/October 1989): 5–9.

26. Though some might argue that such a standard may be a necessary but not sufficient condition of adequate disclosure, my appeal to the transparency model serves as a powerful and therefore useful contrast to physician unilateral decision making.

27. Imbus and Zawacki, "Autonomy for Burned Patients"; Murphy, "Do-Not-Resuscitate Orders."

28. Amir Halevy, Ryan C. Neal, and Baruch A. Brody, "The Low Frequency of Futility in an Adult Intensive Care Unit Setting," *Archives of Internal Medicine* 156 (January 8, 1996): 100–4.

BIBLIOGRAPHY

Books

Applebaum, Paul S., Charles W. Lidz, and Alan Meisel. *Informed Consent: Legal Theory and Clinical Practice*. New York: Oxford University Press, 1987.

Bacon, Francis. *Novum Organum*. Book 1, Aphorism 46.

Barnes, Barry. *Scientific Knowledge and Sociological Theory*. London: Routledge and Kegan Paul, 1974.

Beauchamp, Tom, and James F. Childress. *Principles of Biomedical Ethics*. 3rd ed. New York: Oxford University Press, 1989.

Beauchamp, Tom, and LeRoy Walters, eds. *Contemporary Issues in Bioethics*. 2nd ed. California: Wadsworth Publishing Company, 1982.

Bosk, Charles L. *Forgive and Remember: Managing Medical Failure*. Chicago: University of Chicago Press, 1979.

Brody, Baruch. *Life and Death Decisionmaking*. New York: Oxford University Press, 1988.

Brody, Howard. *The Healer's Power*. New Haven: Yale University Press, 1992.

Callahan, Daniel. *Setting Limits: Medical Goals in an Aging Society*. New York: Simon and Schuster, 1987.

Childress, James F. *Who Should Decide?* New York: Oxford University Press, 1982.

Churchill, Larry R. *Rationing Health Care in America*. Notre Dame: University of Notre Dame Press, 1987.

Code, Lorraine. *What Can She Know? Feminist Theory and the Construction of Knowledge*. Ithaca: Cornell University Press, 1991.

Cranford, Ronald E., and A. Edward Doudera. *Institutional Ethics Committees and Health Care Decisionmaking*. Ann Arbor: AUPHA Press, 1984.

Doudera, A. Edward, and J. Douglas Peters, eds. *Legal and Ethical Aspects of Treating Critically and Terminally Ill Patients*. Ann Arbor: AUPHA Press, 1982.

Dworkin, Gerald, *The Theory and Practice of Autonomy*. Cambridge: Cambridge University Press, 1988.

Eagleton, Terry. *Literary Theory*. Oxford: Blackwell Press, 1985.

Faden, Ruth, and Tom Beauchamp. *A History and Theory of Informed Consent*. New York: Oxford University Press, 1986.

Feinstein, Alvan R. *Clinical Judgment*. Baltimore: Williams and Wilkins, 1967.

Feldman, David. *Health and Medicine in the Jewish Tradition*. New York: Crossroad Publishing, 1986.

Fleck, Ludwik. *Genesis and Development of a Scientific Fact*. 1935 Reprint, Chicago: University of Chicago Press, 1979.

Fried, Charles. *Anatomy of Values*. Cambridge: Harvard University Press, 1970.

164

Harding, Sandra. *The Science Question in Feminism.* Ithaca: Cornell University Press, 1986.

Heisenberg, Werner. *Physics and Philosophy: The Revolution in Modern Science.* New York: Harper and Row, 1958.

——. *Physics and Beyond: Encounters and Conversations.* New York: Harper and Row, 1971.

Hess, Mary. *Revolutions and Reconstructions in the Philosophy of Science.* Bloomington: Indiana University Press, 1980.

Jaggar, Alison M., and Susan R. Bordo, eds. *Gender/Body/Knowledge: Feminist Reconstructions of Being and Knowing.* New Brunswick: Rutgers University Press, 1989.

Jonsen, Albert R., and Stephen Toulmin. *The Abuse of Casuistry.* Berkeley: University of California Press, 1988.

Jonsen, Albert R., Mark Siegler, and Wiliam J. Winslade. *Clinical Ethics: A Practical Approach to Ethical Decisions in Clinical Medicine.* 2nd ed. New York: MacMillan, 1986.

Kass, Leon R. *Toward a More Natural Science: Biology and Human Affairs.* New York: Free Press, 1985.

Katz, Jay. *The Silent World of Doctor and Patient.* New York: Free Press, 1984.

Keller, Evelyn Fox. *Reflections on Gender and Science.* New Haven: Yale University Press, 1985.

Kelly, Gerald. *Medico Moral Problems.* St. Louis: Catholic Hospital Association, 1958.

Kuhn, Thomas. *The Structure of Scientific Revolutions.* 2nd ed. Chicago: University of Chicago Press, 1970.

Latour, Bruno, and Steve Woolgar. *Laboratory Life: The Social Construction of Scientific Facts.* Beverly Hills: Sage, 1979.

Laudan, Larry. *Science and Values.* Berkeley: University of California Press, 1984.

Longino, Helen E. *Science as Social Knowledge: Values and Objectivity in Scientific Inquiry.* Princeton: Princeton University Press, 1990.

Lynn, Joanne, ed. *By No Extraordinary Means: The Choice To Forgo Life-Sustaining Food and Water.* Bloomington: Indiana University Press, 1989.

MacKinnon, Catharine. *Feminism Unmodified.* Cambridge: Harvard University Press, 1987.

McCormick, Richard A., S.J. *Notes on Moral Theology: 1965–1980.* Lanham, Maryland: University Press of America, 1981.

Megill, Allan, ed. *Rethinking Objectivity.* Durham: Duke University Press, 1994.

Meyers, Greg. *Writing Biology.* Madison: University of Wisconsin Press, 1990.

Millman, Marcia. *The Unkindest Cut: Life in the Backrooms of Medicine.* New York: Morrow Quill, 1977.

Moreno, Jonathan D. *Deciding Together: Bioethics and Moral Consensus.* New York: Oxford University Press, 1995.

Morreim, E. Haavi. *Balancing Act: The New Medical Ethics of Medicine's New Economics.* Washington, D.C.: Georgetown University Press, 1995.

Nagel, Thomas. *The View from Nowhere.* New York: Oxford University Press, 1986.

Paget, Marianne A. *The Unity of Mistakes: A Phenomenological Interpretation of Medical Work.* Philadelphia: Temple University Press, 1988.

———. *A Complex Sorrow.* Ed. Marjorie L. DeVault. Philadelphia: Temple University Press, 1993.

Pellegrino, Edmund D., and David C. Thomasma. *A Philosophical Basis of Medical Practice: Toward a Philosophy and Ethic of the Healing Professions.* New York: Oxford University Press, 1981.

———. *For the Patient's Good: The Restoration of Beneficence in Health Care.* New York: Oxford University Press, 1988.

———. *The Virtues in Medical Practice.* New York: Oxford University Press, 1993.

Pincus, Gregory. *The Control of Fertility.* New York: Academic Press, 1965.

Plato. *Republic.* Book 3, 407 c–e.

Ramsey, Paul. *The Patient as Person: Explorations in Medical Ethics.* New Haven: Yale University Press, 1976.

Rawls, John. *A Theory of Justice.* Cambridge: Harvard University Press, 1971.

Rodwin, Marc A. *Medicine, Money, and Morals: Physicians' Conflicts of Interest.* New York: Oxford University Press, 1993.

Rorty, Richard. *Philosophy and the Mirror of Nature.* Princeton: Princeton University Press, 1979.

Schneiderman, Lawrence J., and Nancy S. Jecker. *Wrong Medicine: Doctors, Patients, and Futile Treatment.* Baltimore: Johns Hopkins University Press, 1995.

Stanley, Liz, and Sue Wise. *Breaking Out: Feminist Consciousness and Feminist Research.* London: Routledge and Kegan Paul, 1983.

Veatch, Robert M. *Value-Freedom in Science and Technology.* Missoula, Montana: Scholar's Press: 1976.

———. *Death, Dying and the Biological Revolution.* New Haven: Yale University Press, 1976; rev. ed., 1989.

———. *A Theory of Medical Ethics.* New York: Basic Books, 1981.

———. *The Patient-Physician Relation: The Patient as Partner, Part 2.* Bloomington: Indiana University Press, 1991.

Weir, Robert F. *Abating Treatment With Critically Ill Patients.* New York: Oxford University Press, 1989.

Yankelovich, Daniel. *Coming to Public Judgment: Making Democracy Work in a Complex World.* Syracuse: Syracuse University Press, 1991.

Zoloth-Dorfman, Laurie. "Community and Conscience: The Language of Justice and the Ethics of Health Care Reform." Ph.D. diss., Graduate Theological Union, 1993.

———. *The Ethics of Encounter.* Chapel Hill: University of North Carolina Press, in press.

Zucker, Marjorie B., and Howard D. Zucker, eds. *Medical Futility: And the Evaluation of Life-Sustaining Interventions.* Cambridge, Cambridge University Press, 1997.

Journal Articles

Ackerman, Felicia. "The Significance of a Wish." *Hastings Center Report* 21 (July/August 1991): 27–29.

Ackerman, Terrence J. "Futility Judgments and Therapeutic Conversation." *Journal of the American Geriatrics Society* 42 (August 1994): 902–3.

Alpers, Ann, and Bernard Lo. "Futility: Not Just a Medical Issue." *Law, Medicine, and Health Care* 20 (Winter 1992): 327–29.

———. "When Is CPR Futile?" *Journal of the American Medical Association* 273 (January 11, 1995): 156–58.

Altman, Lawrence K. "Antimicrobial Drugs Endorsed for Ulcers in a Major U.S. Shift." *New York Times* (February 10, 1994): A1, C18.

———. "Stomach Microbe Offers Clues to Cancers as Well as Ulcers." *New York Times* (February 22, 1994): B6.

Amundsen, Darrel W. "The Physician's Obligation to Prolong Life: A Medical Duty Without Classical Roots." *Hastings Center Report* 8 (August 1978): 23–30.

Angell, Marcia. "Respecting the Autonomy of Competent Patients." *New England Journal of Medicine* 310 (April 26, 1984): 1115–16.

———. "The Case of Helga Wanglie: A New Kind of 'Right to Die' Case." *New England Journal of Medicine* 325 (August 15, 1991): 511–12.

Annas, George J. "CPR: When the Beat Should Stop." *Hastings Center Report* 12 (October 1982): 30–31.

Areen, Judith. "The Legal Status of Consent Obtained From Families of Adult Patients to Withhold or Withdraw Treatment." *Journal of the American Medical Association* 258 (July 10, 1987) 229–335.

Asch, David A., John Hansen-Flaschen, and Paul Lanken. "Decisions to Limit or Continue Life-Sustaining Treatment by Critical Care Physicians in the United States: Conflicts between Physicians' Practices and Patients' Wishes." *American Journal of Respiratory and Critical Care Medicine* 151 (February 1995): 288–92.

Bartholome, William G. "Do Not Resuscitate Orders: Accepting Responsibility." *Archives of Internal Medicine* 148 (November 1988): 2345–46.

Bedell, Susanna E. "Survival after Cardiopulmonary Resuscitation in the Hospital." *New England Journal of Medicine* 309 (September 8, 1983): 569–76.

Bedell, Susanna E., and Thomas Delbanco. "Choices About Cardiopulmonary Resuscitation in the Hospital: When Do Physicians Talk With Patients?" *New England Journal of Medicine* 310 (April 26, 1984): 1089–93.

Bedell, Susanna E., et al. "Do-Not-Resuscitate Orders for Critically Ill Patients in the Hospital: How Are They Used and What Is Their Impact?" *Journal of the American Medical Association* 256 (July 11, 1986): 233–37.

Belkin, Lisa. "As Family Protests, Hospital Seeks An End to Woman's Life Support." *New York Times* (January 10, 1991): A1, A16.

Besdine, R. W. "Decisions to Withhold Treatment from Nursing Home Residents." *Journal of the American Geriatric Society* 31 (1983): 602–6.

Blackhall, Leslie J. "Must We Always Use CPR?" *New England Journal of Medicine* 317 (November 12, 1987): 1281–84.

———. "Low Survival Rate After Cardiopulmonary Resuscitation in a County Hospital." *Archives of Internal Medicine* 152 (October 1992): 2045–48.

Brennan, Troyen A. "Do-Not-Resuscitate Orders For the Incompetent Patient in the

Absence of Family Consent." *Law, Medicine, and Health Care* 14 (February 1986): 13–19.

——. "Ethics Committees and Decisions to Limit Care: The Experience at the Massachusetts General Hospital." *Journal of the American Medical Association* 260 (August 12, 1988): 803–7.

——. "Incompetent Patients With Limited Care in the Absence of Family Consent: A Study of Socioeconomic and Clinical Variables." *Annals of Internal Medicine* 109 (November 15, 1988): 819–25.

——. "Silent Decisions: Limits of Consent and the Terminally Ill Patient." *Law, Medicine, and Health Care* 16 (Fall/Winter 1988): 204–9.

Brett, Allan S., and Laurence B. McCullough. "When Patients Request Specific Interventions: Defining the Limits of the Physician's Obligation." *New England Journal of Medicine* 315 (November 20, 1986): 1347–51.

Brock, Dan W., and Steven A. Wartman. "When Competent Patients Make Irrational Choices." *New England Journal of Medicine* 322 (May 31, 1990): 1595–99.

Brockway, George M. "The Physician's Appeal to Firsthand Experience." *Hastings Center Report* 6 (April 1976): 9–12.

Brody, Baruch A., and Amir Halevy. "Is Futility a Futile Concept?" *Journal of Medicine and Philosophy* 20 (April 1995): 123–44.

Brody, Howard. "Transparency: Informed Consent in Primary Care." *Hastings Center Report* 19 (September/October 1989): 5–9.

——. "The Physician's Role in Determining Futility." *Journal of the American Geriatrics Society* 42 (August 1994): 875–78.

Brophy, James M., and Lawrence Joseph. "Placing Trials in Context Using Bayesian Analysis." *Journal of the American Medical Association* 273 (March 15, 1995): 871–75.

Brunetti, Louis L. "Cardiopulmonary Resuscitation Policies and Practices." *Archives of Internal Medicine* 150 (January 1990): 121–26.

Buchanan, Allen. "Medical Paternalism." *Journal of Philosophy and Public Affairs* 7 (Summer 1978): 370–90.

Callahan, Daniel. "Medical Futility, Medical Necessity: The-Problem-Without-A-Name." *Hastings Center Report* 21 (July/August 1991): 30–35.

——. "Necessity, Futility, and the Good Society." *Journal of the American Geriatrics Society* 42 (August 1994): 866–67.

Capron, Alexander M. "Abandoning a Waning Life." *Hastings Center Report* 25 (July/August 1995): 24–26.

Carter, Brian S. and Julie Sandling. "Decision Making in the NICU: The Question of Medical Futility." *The Journal of Clinical Ethics* 3 (Summer 1992): 142–43.

Cassell, Eric J. "The Function of Medicine." *Hastings Center Report* 7 (December 1977): 16–19.

——. "The Nature of Suffering and the Goals of Medicine." *New England Journal of Medicine* 306 (March 10, 1982): 639–45.

Charlson, Mary E. "Resuscitation: How Do We Decide? A Prospective Study of Physicians' Preferences and the Clinical Course of Hospitalized Patients." *Journal of the American Medical Association* 255 (March 14, 1986): 1316–22.

Charlson, Mary E., et al. "Assessing Illness Severity: Does Clinical Judgment Work?" *Journal of Chronic Diseases* 39 (June 1986): 439–52.

Chassin, Mark R. "Costs and Outcomes of Medical Intensive Care." *Medical Care* 20 (February 1982): 165–79.

Chipman, Clark, Robert Adelman, and Gary Sexton. "Criteria for Cessation of CPR in the Emergency Department." *Annals of Emergency Medicine* 10 (January 1981): 11–17.

Chu, Daniel Y. "Predicting Survival in AIDS Patients with Respiratory Failure: Application of the APACHE-II Scoring System." *Critical Care Clinics* 9 (January 1993): 89–105.

Code, Lorraine. "Who Cares? The Poverty of Objectivism for a Moral Epistemology." In Megill. 179–95.

Crane, Diana. "Decisions to Treat Critically Ill Patients: A Comparison of Social versus Medical Considerations." *Milbank Memorial Fund Quarterly* 53 (Winter 1975): 1–33.

Cranford, Ronald E. "The Persistent Vegetative State: The Medical Reality (Getting the Facts Straight)." *Hastings Center Report* 18 (February/March 1988): 27–32.

———. "Futility: A Concept in Search of a Definition." *Law, Medicine, and Health Care* 20 (Winter 1992): 307–9.

———. "Medical Futility: Transforming a Clinical Concept into Legal and Social Policies." *Journal of the American Geriatrics Society* 42 (August 1994): 894–98.

Crawshaw, Ralph, Michael Garland, and Brian Hines. "Oregon Health Decisions: An Experiment with Informed Community Consent." *Journal of the American Medical Association* 254 (December 13, 1985): 3213–16.

Cummins, Richard O., and Mickey S. Eisenberg. "Prehospital Cardiopulmonary Resuscitation: Is It Effective?" *Journal of the American Medical Association* 253 (April 26, 1985): 2408–12.

Curtis, Randall J., et al. "Use of the Medical Futility Rationale in Do-Not-Attempt-Resuscitation Orders." *Journal of the American Medical Association* 273 (January 11, 1995): 124–28.

Daniels, Norman. "Why Saying No to Patients in the United States Is So Hard: Cost Containment, Justice, and Provider Autonomy." *New England Journal of Medicine* 314 (May 22, 1986): 1380–83.

Danis, Marion, et al. "A Comparison of Patient, Family, and Nurse Evaluations of the Usefulness of Intensive Care." *Critical Care Medicine* 15 (February 1987): 138–43.

Danis, Marion, et al. "A Comparison of Patient, Family, and Physician Assessments of the Value of Medical Intensive Care." *Critical Care Medicine* 16 (June 1988): 594–600.

Danis, Marion, et al. "Patients' and Families' Preferences for Medical Intensive Care." *Journal of the American Medical Association* 260 (August 12, 1988): 797–802.

"Death of Baby K Leaves a Legacy of Legal Precedents." *Washington Post* (April 7, 1995): B3.

Detsky, Allen S., et al. "Prognosis, Survival and the Expenditure of Hospital Resources for Patients in an Intensive Care Unit." *New England Journal of Medicine* 305 (September 17, 1981): 667–72.

Diamond, George A., and Timothy A. Denton, "Alternative Perspectives on the Biased Foundations of Medical Technology Assessment." *Annals of Internal Medicine* 118 (March 15, 1993): 455–64.

Dobkin, Jack E., and Ralph E. Cutler. "Use of APACHE-II Classification to Evaluate Outcome of Patients Receiving Hemodialysis in an Intensive Care Unit." *Western Journal of Medicine* 149 (November 1988): 547–50.

Dougherty, Charles J. "Setting Health Care Priorities." Special supplement. *Hastings Center Report* 21 (May/June 1991): 1–10.

Eddy, David M. "What Do We Do About Costs?" *Journal of the American Medical Association* 264 (September 5, 1990): 1161–70.

Edwards, Barbara S. "Withdrawal of Life Support against Family Wishes: Is It Justified? A Case Study." *The Journal of Clinical Ethics* 1 (Spring 1990): 74–79.

Eisenberg, John M. "Sociologic Influences on Decision-Making by Clinicians." *Annals of Internal Medicine* 90 (June 1979): 957–64.

Elstein, Arthur S. "Clinical Judgment: Psychological Research and Medical Practice." *Science* 194 (November 1976): 696–700.

Emanuel, Ezekiel J. "Rights and Responsibilities of Patients and Physicians." In Beauchamp and Walters. 132–41.

———. "A Review of the Ethical and Legal Aspects of Terminating Care." *American Journal of Medicine* 84 (February 1988): 291–301.

Epstein, Arnold M. "The Outcomes Movement—Will It Get Us Where We Want to Go?" *New England Journal of Medicine* 323 (July 26, 1990): 266–70.

Evidence-Based Medicine Working Group. "Evidence-Based Medicine: A New Approach to Teaching the Practice of Medicine." *Journal of the American Medical Association* 268 (November 4, 1992): 2420–25.

Faber-Langendoen, Kathy. "Resuscitation of Patients with Metastatic Cancer: Is Transient Benefit Futile?" *Archives of Internal Medicine* 151 (February 1991): 235–39.

Farber, Neil J., et al. "Cardiopulmonary Resuscitation (CPR): Patient Factors and Decision Making." *Archives of Internal Medicine* 144 (November 1984): 2229–32.

Fee, Elizabeth. "Women's Nature and Scientific Objectivity." In *Women's Nature: Rationalizations of Inequality.* Ed. Marian Lowe and Ruth Hubbard. New York: Pergamon, 1983.

Feinstein, Alvan R. "*Clinical Judgment* Revisited: The Distraction of Quantitative Models." *Annals of Internal Medicine* 120 (May 1994): 799–805.

Fiel, Stanley B. "Heart-Lung Transplantation for Patients With Cystic Fibrosis: A Test of Clinical Wisdom." *Archives of Internal Medicine* 151 (May 1991): 870–72.

Fins, Joseph J., special editor. Futility in Clinical Practice Series. "Futility in Clinical Practice: Report on a Congress of Clinical Societies." *Journal of the American Geriatrics Society* 42 (August 1994): 861–65.

Forrow, Lachlan, Steven Wartman, and Dan Brock. "Science, Ethics, and the Making of Clinical Decisions: Implications for Risk Factor Intervention." *Journal of the American Medical Association* 259 (June 3, 1988): 3161–67.

Franklin, Cory, et al. "Triage Considerations in Medical Intensive Care." *Archives of Internal Medicine* 150 (July 1990): 1455–59.

"Futility: Using SUPPORT to GUIDe Our Fix on Futility." *Hospital Ethics* 11 (January/February 1995): 1–5.

Garland, Michael. "Justice, Politics, and Community: Expanding Access and Rationing Health Services in Oregon." *Law, Medicine, and Health Care* 20 (Spring/Summer 1992): 67–72.

Gatter, Robert A., and John C. Moskop. "From Futility to Triage." *Journal of Medicine and Philosophy* 20 (April 1995): 191–205.

George, Alfred L., et al. "Pre-Arrest Morbidity and Other Correlates of Survival after In-Hospital Cardiopulmonary Arrest." *American Journal of Medicine* 87 (July 1989): 28–34.

Gold, Jay A., et al. "Is There A Right to Futile Treatment? The Case of a Dying Patient With AIDS." *The Journal of Clinical Ethics* 1 (Spring 1990): 19–23.

Gordon, Michael, and Eric Hurovwitz. "Cardiopulmonary Resuscitation of the Elderly." *Journal of the American Geriatric Society* 32 (December 1984): 930–34.

Gorovitz, Samuel, and Alasdair MacIntyre. "Toward a Theory of Medical Fallibility." *Journal of Medicine and Philosophy* 1 (March 1976): 51–71.

Grant, Edward R. "Medical Futility: Legal and Ethical Aspects." *Law, Medicine, and Health Care* 20 (Winter 1992): 330–39.

Gray, William A., Robert J. Capone, and Albert S. Most. "Unsuccessful Emergency Medical Resuscitation—Are Continued Efforts in the Emergency Department Justified?" *New England Journal of Medicine* 325 (November 14, 1991): 1393–98.

Griener, Glenn G. "The Physician's Authority to Withhold Futile Treatment." *Journal of Medicine and Philosophy* 20 (April 1995): 207–224.

Grimes, David A. "Technological Follies: The Uncritical Acceptance of Medical Innovation." *Journal of the American Medical Association* 269 (June 16, 1993): 3030–33.

Gross, Peter A. "Comparison of Severity of Illness Indicators in an Intensive Care Unit." *Archives of Internal Medicine* 151 (November 1991): 2201–5.

Hackler, Chris J., and Charles F. Hiller. "Family Consent to Orders Not to Resuscitate: Reconsidering Hospital Policy." *Journal of the American Medical Association* 264 (September 12, 1990): 1281–83.

Halevy, Amir, and Baruch A. Brody. "A Multi-institutional Collaborative Policy on Medical Futility." *Journal of the American Medical Association* 276 (August 21, 1996): 571–74.

Halevy, Amir, Ryan C. Neal, and Baruch A. Brody. "The Low Frequency of Futility in an Adult Intensive Care Unit Setting." *Archives of Internal Medicine* 156 (January 8, 1996): 100–4.

Hammond, Jeffrey, and C. Gillon Ward. "Decision Not To Treat: 'Do Not Resuscitate' Order for the Burn Patient in the Acute Setting." *Critical Care Medicine* 17 (February 1989): 136–38.

Hansen-Flaschen, John H. "When Life Support is Futile." *Chest* 100 (November 1991): 1191–92.

Haraway, Donna. "Situated Knowledges: The Science Question in Feminism and the Privilege of Partial Perspective." *Feminist Studies* 14 (Fall 1988): 575–99.

Hardwig, John. "Treating the Brain Dead for the Benefit of the Family." *Journal of Clinical Ethics* 2 (Spring 1991): 53–56.

Hawkesworth, Mary E. "From Objectivity to Objectification." In Megill. 151–177.

Hippocrates. "The Art." In *Hippocrates*. Vol. 2. Trans. W. H. S. Jones. Loeb Classical Library. Cambridge: Harvard University Press, 1967. 185–217.

Hosking, Michael P., et al. "Outcomes of Surgery in Patients 90 Years of Age and Older." *Journal of the American Medical Association* 261 (April 17, 1989): 1909–15.

"Hospitals Establish Policies to Limit Futile Care." *Hospital Ethics* 9 (September/October 1993): 10–12.

Howe, Edmund G. "Discussing Futility." *Journal of Clinical Ethics* 5 (Summer 1994): 91–99.

Hudson, Teresa. "Are Futile-Care Policies the Answer?" *Hospitals and Health Networks* 68 (February 20, 1994) 26–32.

Hunter, Kathryn Montgomery. "There Was This One Guy . . . : The Uses of Anecdotes in Medicine." *Perspectives in Biology and Medicine* 29 (Summer 1986): 619–30.

Hyman, David A. "Aesthetics and Ethics: The Implications of Cosmetic Surgery." *Perspectives in Biology and Medicine* 33 (Winter 1990): 190–202.

Imbus, Sharon H., and Bruce E. Zawacki. "Autonomy for Burned Patients When Survival is Unprecedented." *New England Journal of Medicine* 297 (August 11, 1977): 308–11.

Ingelfinger, Franz. "Arrogance." *New England Journal of Medicine* 303 (December 25, 1980): 1507–11.

Jackson, David L., and Stuart Youngner. "Patient Autonomy and Death With Dignity." *New England Journal of Medicine* 301 (August 23, 1979): 404–8.

Jecker, Nancy S. "Knowing When to Stop: The Limits of Medicine." *Hastings Center Report* 21 (May/June 1991): 5–8.

———. "Calling It Quits: Stopping Futile Treatment and Caring for Patients." *Journal of Clinical Ethics* 5 (Summer 1994): 138–42.

———. "Is Refusal of Futile Treatment Unjustified Paternalism?" *Journal of Clinical Ethics* 6 (Summer 1995): 133–37.

Jecker, Nancy S., and Robert A. Pearlman. "Medical Futility: Who Decides?" *Archives of Internal Medicine* 152 (June 1992): 1140–44.

Jecker, Nancy S., and Lawrence J. Schneiderman. "Futility and Rationing." *American Journal of Medicine* 92 (February 1992): 189–96.

———. "Ceasing Futile Resuscitation in the Field: Ethical Considerations." *Archives of Internal Medicine* 152 (December 1992): 2392–97.

———. "An Ethical Analysis of the Use of 'Futility' in the 1992 American Heart Association Guidelines for Cardiopulmonary Resuscitation and Emergency Cardiac Care." *Archives of Internal Medicine* 153 (October 11, 1993): 2195–98.

———. "When Families Request That "Everything Possible" Be Done." *Journal of Medicine and Philosophy* 20 (April 1995): 145–163.

Jennings, Bruce. "A Grassroots Movement in Bioethics." Special supplement. *Hastings Center Report* 18 (June/July 1988): 1–16.

Jennings, Bruce, et al. "Grassroots Bioethics Revisited: Health Care Priorities and Community Values." Special issue. *Hastings Center Report* 20 (September/October 1990): 16–23.

Johnson White, Linda. "Clinical Uncertainty, Medical Futility and Practice Guidelines." *Journal of the American Geriatrics Society* 42 (August 1994): 899–901.

Jonsen, Albert R. "Do No Harm." *Annals of Internal Medicine* 88 (June 1978): 827–32.

——. "What Does Life Support Support?" *Pharos* 50 (1987): 4–7.

——. "Intimations of Futility." *American Journal of Medicine* 96 (February 1994): 107–9.

Kapp, Marshall B. "Futile Medical Treatment: A Review of the Ethical Arguments and Legal Holdings." *Journal of General Internal Medicine* 9 (March 1994): 170–77.

Kass, Leon R. "Ethical Dilemmas in the Care of the Ill, II: What is the Patient's Good?" *Journal of the American Medical Association* 244 (October 24/31, 1980): 1946–49.

Kassirer, Jerome P. "Adding Insult to Injury: Usurping Patients' Prerogatives." *New England Journal of Medicine* 308 (April 14, 1983): 898–901.

Kellermann, Arthur L., et al. "In-Hospitalization Resuscitation Following Unsuccessful Prehospital Advanced Cardiac Life Support: 'Heroic Efforts' Or an Exercise in Futility?" *Annals of Emergency Medicine* 17 (June 1988): 589–94.

Kilner, John F. "Ethical Issues in the Initiation and Termination of Treatment." *American Journal of Kidney Disease* 15 (March 1990): 218–27.

Knaus, William A., and David B. Nash. "Predicting and Evaluating Patient Outcomes." *Annals of Internal Medicine* 109 (October 1988): 521–22.

Knaus, William A., Douglas P. Wagner, and Joanne Lynn. "Short-Term Mortality Predictions for Critically Ill Hospitalized Adults: Science and Ethics." *Science* 254 (October 18, 1991): 389–94.

Knaus, William A., et al. "APACHE II: A Severity of Disease Classification System." *Critical Care Medicine* 13 (October 1985): 818–29.

——. "Prognosis in Acute Organ-System Failure." *Annals of Surgery* 202 (December 1985): 685–93.

Knaus, William A., et al. "The APACHE III Prognostic System: Risk Prediction of Hospital Mortality for Critically Ill Hospitalized Adults." *Chest* 100 (December 1991): 1619–36.

Knaus, William A., et al. "The SUPPORT Prognostic Model: Objective Estimates of Survival for Seriously Ill Hospitalized Adults." *Annals of Internal Medicine* 122 (February 1995): 191–203.

Koch, Kathryn A., Bruce W. Meyers, and Stephen Sandroni. "Analysis of Power in Medical Decision-Making: An Argument for Physician Autonomy." *Law, Medicine, and Health Care* 20 (Winter 1992): 320–26.

Kodish, Eric, et al. "Bone Marrow Transplantation for Sickle Cell Disease: A Study of Parents' Decisions." *New England Journal of Medicine* 325 (November 7, 1991): 1349–53.

Kolata, Gina. "Heart Study Reports Early Revival Is Key to Surviving Attack." *New York Times* (November 14, 1991): A1, A11.

———. "Withholding Care From Patients: Boston Case Asks, Who Decides?" *New York Times* (April 3, 1995): A1, C10.

———. "Court Ruling Limits Rights of Patients: Care Deemed Futile May Be Withheld." *New York Times* (April 22, 1995): A6.

Kopelman, Loretta M. "Conceptual and Moral Disputes about Futile and Useful Treatments." *Journal of Medicine and Philosophy* 20 (April 1995): 109–21.

Korenbrot, Carol. "Experiences With Systemic Contraceptives." In *Toxic Substances: Decisions and Values, Conference II: Information Flow.* Washington, D.C.: Technical Information Project, 1979. 11–42.

Landry, Francis J., Joseph M. Parker, and Yancy Y. Phillips. "Outcome of Cardiopulmonary Resuscitation in the Intensive Care Setting." *Archives of Internal Medicine* 152 (November 1992): 2305–08.

Lantos, John D. "Futility Assessments and the Doctor-Patient Relationship." *Journal of the American Geriatrics Society* 42 (August 1994): 868–70.

Lantos, John D., et al. "Survival After Cardiopulmonary Resuscitation in Babies of Very Low Birth Weight: Is CPR Futile Therapy?" *New England Journal of Medicine* 318 (January 14, 1988): 91–95.

Lantos, John D., et al. "The Illusion of Futility in Clinical Practice." *American Journal of Medicine* 87 (July 1989): 81–84.

La Puma, John, et al. "The Standard of Care: A Case Report and Ethical Analysis." *Annals of Internal Medicine* 108 (January 1988): 121–24.

Laupacis, Andreas, et al. "An Assessment of Clinically Useful Measures of the Consequences of Treatment." *New England Journal of Medicine* 318 (June 30, 1988): 1728–33.

Lawrence Valerie A., and Gary M. Clark. "Cancer and Resuscitation: Does the Diagnosis Affect the Decision?" *Archives of Internal Medicine* 147 (September 1987): 1637–40.

Leikin, Sanford. "When Parents Demand Treatment." *Pediatric Annals* 18 (April 1989): 266–68.

Letter to the editor. "Do Not Resuscitate Orders." *Journal of the American Medical Association* 255 (June 13, 1986): 3114–15.

———. "Ethics of Life Support and Resuscitation." *New England Journal of Medicine* 318 (June 30, 1988): 1754–58.

———. "Reappraisal of DNR Orders in Long-Term-Care Institutions." *Journal of the American Medical Association* 261 (March 17, 1989): 1582–83.

———. "Decision Making in 'Near Death.' " *New England Journal of Medicine* 322 (May 31, 1990): 1604–6.

———. "The Case of Baby L." *New England Journal of Medicine* 323 (October 18, 1990): 1148–49.

———. "Medical Futility." *Annals of Internal Medicine* 114 (January 15, 1991): 169–70.

———. "Family Consent to Orders Not to Resuscitate." *Journal of the American Medical Association* 265 (January 16, 1991): 354–56.

——. "Questions About DNR Orders." *Journal of the American Medical Association* 266 (August 14, 1991): 794–95.

——. "Futility as a Criterion in Limiting Treatment." *New England Journal of Medicine* 327 (October 22, 1992): 1239–41.

——. "The Houston City Wide Policy on Medical Futility." *Journal of the American Medical Association* 276 (November 20, 1996): 1549–50.

Levine, George. "Why Science Isn't Literature." In Megill. 65–79.

Levy, David E., et al. "Predicting Outcome From Hypoxic-Ischemic Coma." *Journal of the American Medical Association* 253 (March 8, 1985): 1420–26.

Lindemann Nelson, James. "Families and Futility." *Journal of the American Geriatrics Society* 42 (August 1994): 879–82.

Lo, Bernard. "The Death of Clarence Herbert: Withdrawing Care Is Not Murder." *Annals of Internal Medicine* 101 (August 1984): 248–51.

——. "Life-sustaining Treatment in Patients with AIDS." In *The Meaning of AIDS: Vol I.* Ed. Eric T. Juengst and Barbara A. Koenig. New York: Praeger, 1989. 86–93.

——. "Unanswered Questions About DNR Orders." *Journal of the American Medical Association* 265 (April 10, 1991): 1874–75.

Lo, Bernard, and Albert R. Jonsen. "Clinical Decisions to Limit Treatment." *Annals of Internal Medicine* 93 (November 1980): 764–68.

Lo, Bernard, and Robert L. Steinbrook. "Deciding Whether to Resuscitate." *Archives of Internal Medicine* 143 (August 1983): 1561–63.

Lo, Bernard, Gary A. McLeod, and Glenn Saika. "Patient Attitudes to Discussing Life-Sustaining Treatment." *Archives of Internal Medicine* 146 (August 1986): 1613–15.

Luce, John M. "Physicians Do Not Have a Responsibility to Provide Futile or Unreasonable Care if a Patient or Family Insists." *Critical Care Medicine* 23 (April 1995): 760–66.

Luce, John M., Robert M. Wachter, and Philip C. Hopewell. "Intensive Care of Patients with the Acquired Immunodeficiency Syndrome: Time for a Reassessment?" *American Review of Respiratory Disease* 137 (June 1988): 1261–63.

Lynn, Joanne, and David DeGrazia. "An Outcomes Model of Medical Decision Making." *Theoretical Medicine* 12 (December 1991): 325–43.

Marsh, Frank H., and Allen Staver. "Physician Authority for Unilateral DNR Orders." *Journal of Legal Medicine* 12 (June 1991): 115–65.

Martin, A. R. "Exploring Patient Beliefs: Steps To Enhancing Physician-Patient Interaction." *Archives of Internal Medicine* 143 (September 1983): 1773–75.

McCartney, James J. "The Development of the Doctrine of Ordinary and Extraordinary Means of Preserving Life in Catholic Moral Theology Before the Karen Quinlan Case." *Linacre Quarterly* 47 (1980): 215–24.

McClellan, Mark, Barbara J. McNeil, and Joseph P. Newhouse. "Does More Intensive Treatment of Acute Myocardial Infarction in the Elderly Reduce Mortality? Analysis Using Instrumental Variables." *Journal of the American Medical Association* 272 (September 21, 1994): 859–66.

McCormick, Richard. "To Save or Let Die: The Dilemma of Modern Medicine." *Journal of the American Medical Association* 229 (July 8, 1974): 173–75.

McCrary, S. Van., et al. "Physicians' Quantitative Assessments of Medical Futility." *Journal of Clinical Ethics* 5 (Summer 1994): 100–5.

McIntyre, Kevin M. "Cardiopulmonary Resuscitation in Chronically Ill Patients in the Intensive Care Unit: Does Poor Outcome Justify Withholding Cardiopulmonary Resuscitation From This Group?" *Archives of Internal Medicine* 152 (November 1992): 2181–83.

Merton, Robert K. "Science, Technology and Society in Seventeenth-Century England." *Osiris* 4 (1938): 360–62.

Miles, Steven H. "Futile Feeding at the End of Life: Family Virtues and Treatment Decisions." *Theoretical Medicine* 8 (October 1987): 293–302.

———. "Resuscitating the Nursing Home Resident: Futility and Pseudofutility." *Journal of the American Geriatrics Society* 38 (September 1990): 1037–38.

———. "Informed Demand for 'Non-Beneficial' Medical Treatment." *New England Journal of Medicine* 325 (August 15, 1991): 512–15.

———. "Medical Futility." *Law, Medicine, and Health Care* 20 (Winter 1992): 310–15.

———. "Interpersonal Issues in the Wanglie Case." *Kennedy Institute of Ethics Journal* 2 (March 1992): 61–72.

Miles, Steven H., Peter A. Singer, and Mark Siegler. "Conflicts Between Patients' Wishes To Forgo Treatment and the Policies of Health Care Facilities." *New England Journal of Medicine* 321 (July 6, 1989): 48–50.

Miller, Donna L., et al. "Cardiopulmonary Resuscitation: How Useful? Attitudes and Knowledge of an Elderly Population." *Archives of Internal Medicine* 152 (March 1992): 578–82.

Miller, Ronald B. "Medical Futility: A Value Dependent Concept." *Loma Linda University Center for Christian Bioethics Newsletter* 7 (December 1991): 3–5.

Miller, Franklin G. "The Concept of Medically Indicated Treatment." *Journal of Medicine and Philosophy* 18 (February 1993): 91–98.

Mirvis, David B. "Physicians' Autonomy—The Relation Between Public and Professional Expectations." *New England Journal of Medicine* 328 (May 6, 1993): 1346–1349.

Moore, Francis D. "The Desperate Case: CARE (Costs, Applicability, Research, Ethics.)" *Journal of the American Medical Association* 261 (March 10, 1989): 1483–84.

Moroff, Saul V. "Qualitative and Ethical Issues in Quantitative Clinical Decision Making." *New York State Journal of Medicine* (May 1986): 250–53.

Moss, Alvin H. "Informing the Patient About Cardiopulmonary Resuscitation: When the Risks Outweigh the Benefits." *Journal of General Internal Medicine* 4 (July/August 1989): 349–55.

Murphy, Donald J. "Do-Not-Resuscitate Orders: Time for Reappraisal in Long-Term-Care Institutions." *Journal of the American Medical Association* 260 (October 14, 1988): 2098–2101.

———. "Can We Set Futile Care Policies? Institutional and Systemic Challenges." *Journal of the American Geriatrics Society* 42 (August 1994): 890–93.

Murphy, Donald J., et al. "Outcomes of Cardiopulmonary Resuscitation in the Elderly." *Annals of Internal Medicine* 111 (August 1, 1989): 199–205.

Murphy, Donald J., Gail J. Povar, and L. Gregory Pawlson. "Setting Limits in Clinical Medicine." *Archives of Internal Medicine* 154 (March 14, 1994): 505–11.

Murphy, Donald J., and Elizabeth Barbour. "GUIDe (Guidelines for the Use of Intensive Care Services in Denver): A Community Effort to Define Futile and Inappropriate Treatment." *New Horizons* 2 (August 1994): 326–31.

Murphy, James J. "Beyond Autonomy: Judicial Restraint and the Legal Limits Necessary to Uphold the Hippocratic Tradition and Preserve the Ethical Integrity of the Medical Profession." *Journal of Contemporary Health Law and Policy* 9 (September 1993): 451–84.

Nelson, Lawrence J. "Primum Utilis Esse." *Yale Journal of Biology and Medicine* 51 (1978): 655–67.

Nelson, Lawrence J., and Robert M. Nelson. "Ethics and the Provision of Futile, Harmful, or Burdensome Treatment to Children." *Critical Care Medicine* 20 (March 1992): 427–33.

Niemann, James T. "Cardiopulmonary Resuscitation." Review Article. *New England Journal of Medicine* 327 (October 8, 1992): 1075–80.

Nolan, Kathleen. "In Death's Shadow: The Meanings of Withholding Resuscitation." *Hastings Center Report* 17 (October/November 1987): 9–14.

Olick, Robert S. "Brain Death, Religious Freedom, and Public Policy: New Jersey's Landmark Legislative Initiative." *Kennedy Institute of Ethics Journal* 1 (December 1991): 275–88.

Osborne, Molly L. "Physician Decisions Regarding Life Support in the Intensive Care Unit." *Chest* 101 (January 1992): 222–23.

Paris, John J., and Robert K. Crone. "Physician Refusal of Requests for Futile or Ineffective Interventions." *Cambridge Quarterly of Healthcare Ethics* 2 (1992): 127–34.

Paris, John J., Robert K. Crone, and Frank E. Reardon. "Physicians' Refusal of Requested Treatment: The Case of Baby L." *New England Journal of Medicine* 322 (April 5, 1990): 1012–15.

Paris, John J., et al. "Beyond Autonomy—Physicians' Refusal to Use Life-Prolonging Extracorporeal Membrane Oxygenation." *New England Journal of Medicine* 329 (July 29, 1993): 354–57.

Pearlman, Robert A. "Medical Futility: Where Do We Go From Here?" *Journal of the American Geriatrics Society* 42 (August 1994): 904–5.

Pearlman, Robert A., and Albert R. Jonsen. "The Use of Quality-of-Life Considerations in Medical Decision Making." *Journal of the American Geriatrics Society* 33 (May 1985): 344–52.

Pearlman, Robert A., Thomas S. Inui, and William B. Carter. "Variability in Physician Bioethical Decision-Making: A Case Study of Euthanasia." *Annals of Internal Medicine* 97 (September 1982): 420–25.

Pearlman, Robert A., Richard F. Uhlmann, and Nancy S. Jecker. "Spousal Understanding of Patient Quality of Life: Implications for Surrogate Decision Making." *Journal of Clinical Ethics* 3 (Summer 1992): 114–20.

Pellegrino, Edmund D. "Withholding and Withdrawing Treatments: Ethics at the Bedside." *Clinical-Neurosurgery* 35 (1989): 164–84.

Perkins, Henry S. "Ethics at the End of Life: Practical Principles for Making Resuscitation Decisions." *Journal of General Internal Medicine* 1 (May/June 1986): 170–76.

Perry, Clifton B., and William B. Applegate. "Medical Paternalism and Patient Self-Determination." *Journal of the American Geriatrics Society* 33 (May 1985) 353–59.

Podrid, Philip J. "Resuscitation in the Elderly: A Blessing or a Curse?" *Annals of Internal Medicine* 111 (August 1989): 193–95.

Poses, Roy M. "The Accuracy of Experienced Physicians' Probability Estimates for Patients with Sore Throats: Implications for Decision Making." *Journal of the American Medical Association* 254 (August 16, 1985): 925–29.

———. "The Answer to 'What are my chances, doctor?' Depends on Whom is Asked: Prognostic Disagreement and Inaccuracy for Critically Ill Patients." *Critical Care Medicine* 17 (August 1989): 827–33.

Post, Stephen G. "My Conscience, Your Money: Commmentary." *Hastings Center Report* 25 (September/October 1995): 28–29.

Povar, Gail. "Withdrawing and Withholding Therapy: Putting Ethics Into Practice." *The Journal of Clinical Ethics* 1 (Spring 1990): 50–56.

Prendergast, Thomas J. "Futility and the Common Cold: How Requests for Antibiotics Can Illuminate Care at the End of Life." *Chest* 107 (March 1995): 836–44.

Quill, Timothy E., and Nancy M. Bennett. "The Effects of a Hospital Policy and State Legislation on Resuscitation Orders for Geriatric Patients." *Archives of Internal Medicine* 152 (March 1992): 569–72.

Rabeneck, Linda, Catherine M. Viscoli, and Ralph I. Horwitz. "Problems in the Conduct and Analysis of Randomized Clinical Trials: Are We Getting the Right Answers to the Wrong Questions?" *Archives of Internal Medicine* 152 (March 1992): 507–12.

Ramsey, Paul. "Prolonged Dying: Not Medically Indicated." *Hastings Center Report* 6 (February 1976): 14–17.

"Regulations Seen As Culprit In N.Y. Resuscitation Decisions." *Hospital Ethics* (November/December 1990): 5–6.

Relman, Arnold S. "Assessment and Accountability: The Third Revolution in Medical Care." *New England Journal of Medicine* 319 (November 3, 1988): 1220–22.

Rie, Michael A. "The Limits of A Wish." *Hastings Center Report* 21 (July/August 1991): 24–27.

Rosner, Fred. "Must We Always Offer the Option of CPR?: The Law In New York." *Journal of the American Medical Association* 260 (December 2, 1988): 3129.

Ross, Judith Wilson. "Judgments of Futility: What Should Ethics Committees Be Thinking About?" *Hospital Ethics Committee Forum* 3 (1991): 201–10.

Rouse, Fenella. "Mrs. Wanglie and 'Doctor Knows Best' and Making Decisions for

Those Who Cannot Decide for Themselves: Autonomy in Two Recent Cases."
Cambridge Quarterly of Healthcare Ethics 2 (Spring 1992): 165–68.

Ruark, John E., and Thomas A. Raffin. "Initiating and Withdrawing Life Support:
Principles and Practice in Adult Medicine." *New England Journal of Medicine*
318 (January 7, 1988): 25–30.

Santa Monica Hospital Medical Center. "Futile Care Guidelines." Supplement. *Medical Ethics Advisor* 9 (October 1993).

Schiedermayer, David L. "The Decision to Forgo CPR in the Elderly Patient." *Journal
of the American Medical Association* 260 (October 14, 1988): 2096–97.

Schneiderman, Lawrence J. "The Futility Debate: Effective versus Beneficial Intervention." *Journal of the American Geriatrics Society* 42 (August 1994): 883–86.

Schneiderman, Lawrence J., and Nancy S. Jecker. "Futility in Practice." *Archives of
Internal Medicine* 153 (February 22, 1993): 437–40.

Schneiderman, Lawrence J., and Roger G. Spragg. "Ethical Decisions in Discontinuing Mechanical Ventilation." *New England Journal of Medicine* 318 (April 14,
1988): 984–88.

Schneiderman, Lawrence J., Kathy Faber-Langendoen, and Nancy S. Jecker. "Beyond
Futility to an Ethic of Care." *American Journal of Medicine* 96 (February 1994):
110–14.

Schneiderman, Lawrence J., Nancy S. Jecker, and Albert R. Jonsen. "Medical Futility:
Its Meaning and Ethical Implications." *Annals of Internal Medicine* 15 (June 15,
1990): 949–54.

———. "Medical Futility: Response to Critiques." *Annals of Internal Medicine* 125
(October 15, 1996): 669–74.

Schneiderman, Lawrence J., et al. "Do Physicians' Own Preferences for Life-Sustaining Treatment Influence Their Perceptions of Patients' Preferences?" *Journal of
Clinical Ethics* 4 (Spring 1993): 28–32.

Schoen, Wendy L. Note. "Conflict in the Parameters Defining Life and Death in Missouri Statutes." *American Journal of Law and Medicine* 16 (1990): 555–72.

Schuster, Daniel P., and Jay M. Marion. "Precedents for Meaningful Recovery During Treatment in Medical Intensive Care Units: Outcomes in Patients with Hematologic Malignancy." *American Journal of Medicine* 75 (September 1983):
402–8.

Schwartz, Robert L. "Autonomy, Futility, and the Limits of Medicine." *Cambridge
Quarterly of Healthcare Ethics* 2 (1992): 159–164.

Shankel, Stewart, Chairman. Futile Care Ad Hoc Committee, San Bernadino County
Medical Society. Communication to all area hospital ethics committee chairpersons. (April 19, 1995).

Shapin, Steven. "History of Science and Its Sociological Constructions." *History of
Science* 20 (1982): 157–211.

Shewmon, D. Alan. "Ethics and Brain Death: A Response." *New Scholasticism* 61
(Summer 1987): 321–44.

———. "Caution in the Definition and Diagnosis of Infant Brain Death." In *Medi-*

cal Ethics: A Guide for Health Professionals Ed. John F. Monagle and David C. Thomasma. Maryland: Aspen Press, 1988. 38–57.

——. "Commentary on Guidelines for the Determination of Brain Death in Children." *Annals of Neurology* 24 (December 1988): 789–91.

Siegler, Mark. "The Doctor-Patient Accommodation: A Central Event in Clinical Medicine." *Archives of Internal Medicine* 142 (October 1982): 1899–1902.

——. "Decision-Making Strategy for Clinical-Ethical Problems in Medicine." *Archives of Internal Medicine* 142 (November 1982): 2178–79.

——. "Does Everything Include CPR?" *Hastings Center Report* 12 (October 1982): 28–30.

——. "Physicians' Refusals of Patient Demands: An Application of Medical Discernment." In *In Search of Equity: Health Needs and the Health Care System*. Ed. Ronald Bayer, Arthur L. Caplan, and Norman Daniels. New York: Plenum, 1983. 199–227.

Solomon, Mildred Z. "How Physicians Talk about Futility: Making Words Mean Too Many Things." *Law, Medicine, and Ethics* 21 (Summer 1993): 231–37.

Spielman, Bethany. "Futility and Bargaining Power." *Journal of Clinical Ethics* 6 (Spring 1995): 44–52.

Starr, Jolene T., Robert A. Pearlman, and Richard F. Uhlmann. "Quality of Life and Resuscitation Decisions in Elderly Patients." *Journal of General Internal Medicine* 1 (November/December 1986): 373–79.

Steinbrook, Robert. "Hospital or Family: Who Decides the Right to Die?" *Los Angeles Times* (February 17, 1991): A1, A40, A41.

Stell, Lance K. "Real Futility: Historical Beginnings and Continuing Debate About Futile Treatment." *North Carolina Medical Journal* 56 (September 1995): 432–38.

Stephens, Ronald L. "Do Not Resuscitate Orders: Ensuring the Patient's Participation." *Journal of the American Medical Association* 255 (January 10, 1986): 240–41.

Suber, Daniel G., and William J. Tabor. "Withholding of Life Sustaining Treatment From the Terminally Ill, Incompetent Patient: Who Decides? Part I." *Journal of the American Medical Association* 248 (November 12, 1982): 2250–51.

Suber, Daniel G., and William J. Tabor. "Withholding of Life Sustaining Treatment From the Terminally Ill, Incompetent Patient: Who Decides? Part II." *Journal of the American Medical Association* 248 (November 12, 1982): 2431–32.

Sugarman, Jeremy, guest editor. "A Community Policy on Medical Futility? A Conversation of the North Carolina Community." Special issue. *North Carolina Medical Journal* 56 (September 1995): 411–72.

Sullivan, Ronald. "Queens Hospital Accused of Denial of Care." *New York Times* (March 24, 1984): A17.

Taffet, George E., Thomas A. Teasdale, and Robert J. Luchi. "Inhospital Cardiopulmonary Resuscitation." *Journal of the American Medical Association* 260 (October 14, 1988): 2069–72.

Tanenbaum, Sandra J. "Knowing and Acting in Medical Practice: The Epistemological Politics of Outcomes Research." *Journal of Health Politics, Policy, and Law* 19 (Spring 1994): 27–44.

Teno, Joan M., Donald J. Murphy, Joanne Lynn et al. "Prognosis-Based Futility Guidelines: Does Anyone Win?" *Journal of the American Geriatrics Society* 42 (November 1994): 1202–7.

Thibault, George E., et al. "Medical Intensive Care: Indications, Interventions, and Outcomes." *New England Journal of Medicine* 302 (April 24, 1980): 938–42.

Thomasma, David C. "Beyond Medical Paternalism and Patient Autonomy: A Model of Physician Conscience for the Physician-Patient Relationship." *Annals of Internal Medicine* 98 (February 1983): 243–48.

Thurow, Lester C. "Learning to Say 'No'." *New England Journal of Medicine* 311 (December 13, 1984): 1569–72.

Tomlinson, Tom L., and Howard Brody. "Ethics and Communication in Do-Not-Resuscitate Orders." *New England Journal of Medicine* 318 (January 7, 1988): 43–46.

———. "Futility and the Ethics of Resuscitation." *Journal of the American Medical Association* 264 (September 12, 1990): 1276–80.

Tomlinson, Tom L., and Diane Czlonka. "Futility and Hospital Policy." *Hastings Center Report* 25 (May/June 1995): 28–35.

Toms, Steven A. "Outcome Predictors in the Early Withdrawal of Life Support: Issues of Justice and Allocation for the Severely Brain Injured." *Journal of Clinical Ethics* 4 (Fall 1993): 206–10.

Tong, Rosemarie. "Towards a Just, Courageous, and Honest Resolution of the Futility Debate." *Journal of Medicine and Philosophy* 20 (April 1995): 165–89.

Torian, Lucia V. "Decisions for and against Resuscitation in an Acute Geriatric Medicine Unit Serving the Frail Elderly." *Archives of Internal Medicine* 152 (March 1992): 561–65.

Troug, Robert T. "Beyond Futility." *Journal of Clinical Ethics* 3 (Summer 1992): 143–45.

———. "Progress in the Futility Debate." *Journal of Clinical Ethics* 6 (Summer 1995): 128–32.

Troug, Robert T., Allan S. Brett, and Joel Frader. "The Problem With Futility." *New England Journal of Medicine* 326 (June 4, 1992): 1560–64.

Tversky, Amos, and Daniel Kahneman. "Judgment Under Uncertainty: Heuristics and Biases." *Science* 185 (September 1974): 1124–31.

Uhlmann, Richard F., Robert A. Pearlman, and Kevin C. Cain. "Physicians' and Spouses' Predictions of Elderly Patients' Resuscitation Preferences." *Journal of Gerontology* 43 (September 1988): M115–21.

Urberg, Martin, and Carol Ways. "Survival After Cardiopulmonary Resuscitation for an In-Hospital Cardiac Arrest." *Journal of Family Practice* 25 (July 1987): 41–44.

Valenzuela, Terence D., et al. "Case and Survival Definitions of Out-of-Hospital Cardiac Arrest: Effect on Survival Rate Calculation." *Journal of the American Medical Association* 267 (January 8, 1992): 272–74.

Vawter, Dorle. "Professional Integrity Based Objections to Providing Requested Interventions." Paper presented at the Ninth Annual Bioethics Summer Retreat, Hilton Head Island, South Carolina, June 11–15, 1997.

Veatch, Robert M. "The Generalization of Expertise: Scientific Expertise and Value Judgments." *Hastings Center Report* 1 (1973): 29–40.

———. "An Ethical Framework for Terminal Care Decisions: A New Classification of Patients." *Journal of the American Geriatrics Society* 32 (September 1984): 665–69.

———. "Limits of Guardian Treatment Refusal: A Reasonableness Standard." *American Journal of Law and Medicine* 9 (Winter 1984): 427–68.

———. "Deciding Against Resuscitation: Encouraging Signs and Potential Dangers." *Journal of the American Medical Association* 253 (January 4, 1985): 77–78.

———. "Contemporary Bioethics and the Demise of Modern Medicine." In *The Patient-Physician Relation: The Patient as Partner, Part 2.* 263–79.

———. "Consensus of Expertise: The Role of Consensus of Experts in Formulating Public Policy and Estimating Facts." *Journal of Medicine and Philosophy* 16 (August 1991): 427–45.

———. "Justice and Outcomes Research: The Ethical Limits." *Journal of Clinical Ethics* 4 (Fall 1993): 258–61.

———. "What Counts as Basic Health Care? Private Values and Public Policy." *Hastings Center Report* 24 (May/June 1994): 20–21.

———. "Why Physicians Cannot Determine if Care is Futile." *Journal of the American Geriatrics Society* 42 (August 1994): 871–74.

Veatch, Robert M., and Carol Mason Spicer. "Medically Futile Care: The Role of the Physician in Setting Limits." *American Journal of Law and Medicine* 18 (1992): 15–36.

Veatch, Robert M., and William E. Stempsey. "Incommensurability: Its Implications for the Patient/Physician Relationship." *Journal of Medicine and Philosophy* 20 (June 1995): 253–69.

Wachter, Robert M., et al. "Intensive Care of Patients with the Acquired Immunodeficiency Syndrome: Outcome and Changing Patterns of Utilization." *American Review of Respiratory Diseases* 134 (1986): 891–96.

Wachter, Robert M., et al. "Attitudes of Medical Residents Regarding Intensive Care for Patients With the Acquired Immunodeficiency Syndrome." *Archives of Internal Medicine* 148 (January 1988): 149–52.

Wachter, Robert M., et al. "Decisions about Resuscitation: Inequities among Patients with Different Diseases But Similar Prognoses." *Annals of Internal Medicine* 111 (September 1989): 525–32.

Waisel, David B., and Robert B. Troug. "The Cardiopumonary Resuscitation-Not-Indicated Order: Futility Revisited." *Annals of Internal Medicine* 122 (February 15, 1995): 304–8.

Wanzer, Sidney, et al. "The Physician's Responsibility Toward Hopelessly Ill Patients." *New England Journal of Medicine* 310 (April 12, 1984): 955–59.

Wanzer, Sidney, et al. "The Physician's Responsibility Toward Hopelessly Ill Patients, A Second Look." *New England Journal of Medicine* 320 (March 30, 1989): 844–49.

Weaver, Douglas W. "Resuscitation Outside the Hospital—What's Lacking?" *New England Journal of Medicine* 325 (November 14, 1991): 1437–39.

Weijer, Charles, and Carl Elliot. "Pulling the Plug on Futility." *British Medical Journal* 310 (March 18, 1995): 683–84.

Weiser, Benjamin. "The Case of Baby Rena: Who Decides When Care Is Futile?" *The Washington Post* July 14, 1991.

Wolf, Susan M. "Conflict Between Doctor and Patient." *Law, Medicine, and Health Care* 16 (Fall/Winter 1988): 197–203.

———. " 'Near Death'—In the Moment of Decision." *New England Journal of Medicine* 322 (January 18, 1990): 208–10.

Yarborough, Mark. "Continued Treatment of the Fatally Ill for the Benefit of Others." *Journal of the American Geriatric Society* 36 (January 1988): 63–7.

Youngner, Stuart J. "Do-Not-Resuscitate Orders: No Longer Secret, But Still a Problem." *Hastings Center Report* 17 (February 1987): 24–33.

———. "Who Defines Futility?" *Journal of the American Medical Association* 260 (October 14, 1988): 2094–95.

———. "Futility in Context." *Journal of the American Medical Association* 264 (September 12, 1990): 1295–96.

———. "Applying Futility: Saying No is Not Enough." *Journal of the American Geriatrics Society* 42 (August 1994): 887–89.

Youngner, Stuart J., et al. "Do Not Resuscitate Orders: Incidence and Implications in a Medical Intensive Care Unit." *Journal of American Medical Association* 253 (January 4, 1985): 54–57.

Zawacki, Bruce. "Tongue-Tied in the Burn Intensive Care Unit." *Critical Care Medicine* 17 (1989): 198–99.

———. "The 'Futility Debate' and the Management of Gordian Knots." *Journal of Clinical Ethics* 6 (Summer 1995): 112–27.

Official Documents and Position Papers

Ad hoc Committee of the Harvard Medical School to Examine the Definition of Brain Death. "A Definition of Irreversible Coma." *Journal of the American Medical Association* 205 (August 5, 1968): 337–40.

American Academy of Neurology. "Guidelines on the Vegetative State: Commentary on the American Academy of Neurology Statement and Position of the American Academy of Neurology on Certain Aspects of the Care and Management of the Persistent Vegetative State." *Neurology* 39 (January 1989): 123–26.

American College of Chest Physicians/Society for Critical Care Medicine (ACCP/SCCM) Consensus Panel. "Ethical and Moral Guidelines for the Initiation, Continuation, and Withdrawal of Intensive Care." *Chest* 97 (April 1990): 949–58.

American College of Physicians Ethics Manual. Part 1: "History; The Patient; Other Physicians." *Annals of Internal Medicine* 111 (August 1, 1989): 245–52.

American College of Physicians Ethics Manual. Part 2: "The Physician and Society; Research; Life-Sustaining Treatment; Other Issues." *Annals of Internal Medicine* 111 (August 15, 1989): 327–35.

American College of Physicians Ethics Manual. 3rd ed. U.S.A.: American College of Physicians, 1993.

American Hospital Association. "Policy and Statement: The Patient's Choice of Treatment Options." Chicago: American Hospital Association, 1985.

American Thoracic Society, Medical Section of the American Lung Association. "Withholding and Withdrawing Life-Sustaining Therapy." *American Review of Respiratory Disease* 144 (September 1991): 726–31.

Appleton Consensus. "Suggested International Guidelines for the Initiation, Continuation, and Withdrawal of Intensive Care." *Chest* 97 (1990): 949–58.

Berenson, R. A. *Intensive Care Units (ICUs): Clinical Outcomes, Costs, and Decision Making (Health Technology Case Study 28)* (U.S. Congress OTA-HCS-28). Washington, D.C.: Office of Technology Assessment (November 1984).

Clinical Care Committee of the Massachusetts General Hospital. "Optimum Care for Hopelessly Ill Patients." *New England Journal of Medicine* 295 (August 12, 1976): 362–64.

Congregation for the Doctrine of the Faith. *Declaration On Euthanasia.* Rome: Sacred Congregation for the Doctrine of the Faith, May 5, 1980.

Council on Ethical and Judicial Affairs. "Statement on Withdrawing Life Prolonging Medical Treatment." *Journal of the American Medical Association* 256 (March 15, 1986): 471.

——. "Guidelines for the Appropriate Use of Do-Not-Resuscitate Orders." *Journal of the American Medical Association* 265 (April 10, 1991): 1868–71.

——. *Code of Medical Ethics.* Chicago: American Medical Association, 1994.

Ethics Committee, Society of Critical Care Medicine. "Consensus Statement of the Society of Critical Care Medicine's Ethics Committee Regarding Futile and Other Possibly Inadvisable Treatment." *Critical Care Medicince* 25 (May 1997): 887–91.

The Hastings Center. *Guidelines on the Termination of Life-Sustaining Treatment and the Care of the Dying.* Briarcliff Manor, New York: The Hastings Center, 1987.

Joint Committee on Biomedical Ethics, Los Angeles County Medical Association and Los Angeles County Bar Association. "Guidelines for Forgoing Life-Sustaining Treatment for Adult Patients." *LACMA Physician* 129 (1990): 31–36.

The Linacre Centre. "Prolongation of Life, Paper 3: Ordinary and Extraordinary Means of Prolonging Life." London: *Linacre Centre*, 1979.

National Conference on Cardiopulmonary Resuscitation and Emergency Cardiac Care. "Standards and Guidelines for Cardiopulmonary Resuscitation and Emergency Cardiac Care: Medicolegal Considerations and Recommendations." *Journal of the American Medical Association* 227 (February 18, 1974): 864–65; 244 (August 1, 1980): 511–12; 255 (June 6, 1986): 2979–84.

The New York State Task Force on Life and the Law. *Do Not Resuscitate Orders.* 2nd ed. New York, 1986.

——. "Standards and Guidelines for Cardiopulmonary Resuscitation and Emergency Cardiac Care: Ethical Considerations in Resuscitation." *Journal of the American Medical Association* 268 (October 28, 1992): 2282–88.

Pope Pius XII. "The Prolongation of Life: An Address of Pope Pius XII to an International Congress of Anesthesiologists." *The Pope Speaks* 4 (Spring 1958): 393–98.

President's Commission for the Study of Ethical Problems in Medicine and Biomedical and Behavioral Research. *Defining Death: Medical, Legal and Ethical Issues in the Definition of Death.* Washington, D.C.: U.S. Government Printing Office, July 1981.

President's Commission for the Study of Ethical Problems in Medicine and Biomedical and Behavioral Research. *Making Health Care Decisions: A Report on the Ethical and Legal Implications of Informed Consent in the Patient-Practitioner Relationship.* Washington, D.C.: U.S. Government Printing Office, October 1982.

President's Commission for the Study of Ethical Problems in Medicine and Biomedical and Behavioral Research. *Deciding to Forego Life Sustaining Treatment: A Report on the Ethical, Medical, and Legal Issues in Treatment Decisions.* Washington, D.C.: U.S. Government Printing Office, March 1983.

Task Force on Ethics of the Society of Critical Care Medicine. "Consensus Report on the Ethics of Foregoing Life-Sustaining Treatments in the Critically Ill." *Critical Care Medicine* 18 (1989): 1425–39.

Task Force on Guidelines, Society of Critical Care Medicine. "Recommendations for Intensive Care Unit With Admission and Discharge Criteria." *Critical Care Medicine* 16 (1988): 807–8.

U.S. Congress, Office of Technology Assessment. *Life Sustaining Technologies and the Elderly* (Publication OTA-BA-306). Washington, D.C.: Government Printing Office, 1987.

U.S. Department of Health and Human Services, Office of Human Development Services. "Child Abuse and Neglect Prevention and Treatment." *Federal Register* 50 (April 15, 1985): 14878–88.

Court Cases and Statutes

Article 29-B, Statute 413-A. The State of New York Public Health Law, 1988.

Barber v. Superior Court of California, 147 Cal. App. 3d 1006, 1017–18, 195 Cal. Rptr. 484 (1983).

Bartling v. Superior Court, 163 Cal. App. 3d 186, 209 Cal. Rptr. 220 (1984).

Bouvia V. Superior Court, 225 Cal. R. 297 Cal App. 2d Dis (1986).

Conservatorship of Drabick, 200 Cal. App. 3d. 185 (1988).

Cruzan V. Director, Missouri Department of Health, 110 S.Ct 284 (1990).

Duesning V. Southwest Texas Methodist Hospital, # SA 87 CA 1119, (U.S. District Ct. for the Western District of Texas, San Antonio Division, December 22, 1988).

Gilgunn v. Massachusetts General Hospital, No. 92–4820 (Mass. Sup. Ct. Civ. Action Suffolk Co. April 22, 1995).

In Re Baby K, 832 F. Supp. 1022 (E.D. Va. 1993), *aff'd,* 16 F. 3d 590, (4th Cir. 1994) 16 F. 3d 590, *cert. denied,* 115 S. Ct. 91, 63 U.S.L.W. 3258, 130 L. Ed. 2d 42 (1994).

In Re Quinlan, 70 N.J. 10, 355 A.2d 647, cert. denied sub nom. *Garger v. New Jersey*, 429 U.S. 922 (1976).

Memorandum Issued with Findings of Fact, Conclusions of Law and Order Dated 28 June 1991, *In Re The Conservatorship of Helga M. Wanglie*, # PX-91-282 (District Court Probate Court Division, County of Hennepin, State of Minnesota).

"New Jersey Declaration of Death Act." N.J. Stat. Chs. 26: 6A-8 through 6A-8 (West 1994).

1984 Amendments to the Child Abuse Prevention and Treatment Act. Public Law 98-457, 1984.

Schloendorff V. Society of New York Hospital, 211 N.Y. 125, 105 N.E. 92, 95 (1914).

Superintendent of Belchertown State School v. Saikewicz, 373 Mass. 728, 370 N.E. 2d 417 (1977).

Vacco v. Quill, 138 L. Ed. 2d 834 (1977).

"The Virginia Health Care Decisions Act," Virginia Code, Article 8, 54.1-2990.

Washington v. Glucksberg, 138 L. Ed. 2d 772 (1977).

INDEX

qualitative futility, 57; on uses for statistics, 62, 64; on value choices in physiologic futility judgments, 8, 81, 103
Science: constitutive vs. textual values of,
93; problem of interpretation in, 104–107;
as a social practice, 97, 120; and social values in scientific research, 100–101; uncertainty in, 107–108
Scientific method, 93–94; social constructionist critique of, 103–104; social constructionist model of, 96–98; values embedded in, 99–103
Shewmon, D. Alan, on the determination
of brain death, 101
Social constructionist theory of knowledge,
1, 91, 118; on interpretation, 104–107; on
mistakes, 108–12, 160nn42,47; model for
obtaining scientific knowledge, 96–98; on
objectivity, 95–99; scientific method cri-
tiqued in, 103–104; on uncertainty, 107–
108; on value neutrality, 99–103
Social contract, 120–23, 160n3
Social discourse, 58, 122–25. *See also* Consensus
Society of Critical Care Medicine, 17–18, 22
Spicer, Carol Mason, 121, 132–33
Statistics, use of, 62–65, 155n70
Substituted judgment, standard of, 14
SUPPORT Prognostic Model, 155n70

Theory: antipositivist model of, 98
Thomasma, David C., 80
Tomlinson, Tom L., 22, 49–50, 80, 81, 82
Transparent disclosure, 138–39, 162n26

Treatments: examples of futile treatments,
20; goals of linked to futility judgments,
45–55; ordinary vs. extraordinary, 30, 32;
proportionality test for, 30, 31–33,
149nn53,55; quality of life goals of, 50–52;
relevance of, 127–29; restoration of consciousness goal of, 49–50; temporary use
of futile treatments, 75; traditional goals
of, 48–50. *See also* Futility judgments
Truth: and positivism, 91–92, 157n4

Ulcers: mistakes in treatments for, 109
Uncertainty, problem of, 107–108
Usefulness, criterion of, 30, 31

Values: distinguished from facts, 4–5, 11, 41;
as embedded in scientific practice, 99–
103; normative privileging of factual
judgments over, 5–9, 92; in physiologic futility judgments, 99, 102–103
Vatican: *Declaration on Euthanasia,* 32–33
Veatch, Robert M., 34, 76, 121, 132–33, 155n2;
on the generalization of expertise argument, 34–35, 76–80; on the order of the
principles of bioethics, 155nn75,76; on the
social contract, 160n3

Wanglie, Helga, 24–27, 52, 73, 133–34

Yankelovich, Daniel, 124
Youngner, Stuart, 7, 45, 80

Zawacki, Bruce E., 29, 78, 79
Zoloth-Dorfman, Laurie, 111, 152n32, 155n3

Susan B. Rubin received a doctorate in philosophy and bioethics from The Kennedy Institute of Ethics at Georgetown University and is co-founder of The Ethics Practice, a firm devoted to providing bioethics education, research, and clinical consultation. She has worked as an ethicist in a variety of fee-for-service and managed care settings, including one of the oldest and largest health maintenance organizations in the United States. Rubin has published a number of articles in publications such as *The Journal of Clinical Ethics* and *Theoretical Medicine,* and she is the co-editor of a forthcoming book on mistakes in medicine and ethics consultation.